PLANT
POWERED
PLUS

PLANT POWERED *PLUS*

Activate the Power of Your Gut to Tame
Inflammation and Reclaim Your Health

Will Bulsiewicz, MD

AVERY

an imprint of Penguin Random House
New York

AVERY

an imprint of Penguin Random House LLC
1745 Broadway, New York, NY 10019
penguinrandomhouse.com

Most Avery books are available at a discount when purchased in quantity for sales
promotions or corporate use. Special editions, which include personalized covers, excerpts,
and corporate imprints, can be created when purchased in large quantities. For more
information, please e-mail specialmarkets@penguinrandomhouse.com. Your local bookstore
can also assist with discounted bulk purchases using the Penguin Random House corporate
Business-to-Business program. For assistance in locating a participating retailer, e-mail
B2B@penguinrandomhouse.com.

Book design by Ashley Tucker

Library of Congress Cataloging-in-Publication Data has been applied for.

ISBN 9780593418796
Ebook ISBN 9780593418802

Printed in the United States of America
1st Printing

The authorized representative in the EU for product safety and compliance is Penguin
Random House Ireland, Morrison Chambers, 32 Nassau Street, Dublin D02 YH68, Ireland,
https://eu-contact.penguin.ie.

Dear Mom,

For your fierce loyalty, unwavering dedication to family, and tireless work ethic.

Thank you for sacrificing to create opportunities for my brothers and me, and for modeling the determination that continues to guide me.

I love you, and I'm forever grateful.

This book's for you.

CONTENTS

AUTHOR'S NOTE

If you're holding this book, you're likely searching for answers or seeking a path to better health. Perhaps your own journey has brought you here, or maybe you're hoping to help someone you love. Whatever your reasons, please know that you are in the right place.

Within these pages, you'll discover powerful insights on the critical connection between your gut, inflammation, and your overall health. However, there's something essential you need to hear directly from me: This book is not meant to stand alone. Your health journey should be deeply personal—tailored specifically to your medical history, unique needs, and personal goals.

I urge you to partner with a trusted health care professional. Their guidance will help make sure the strategies and recommendations you find here are safely and effectively personalized to your needs, to help you fulfill your goals.

While I've done my utmost to weave flexibility and personalization into this text, the truth remains: A book is inherently general, written for many. My hope is that even though the words are the same for all, the way that you hear me is unique to you. I hope that you find yourself resonating with these pages.

Before you dive deeper, I encourage you to glance at page 371. There, you'll find a long list of health conditions linked to a damaged gut microbiome, compromised gut barrier, and inflammation. Look closely. If you see multiple items from your health history, you'll know you're in the right place. But you don't need to be sick to benefit from this book. How wonderful would it be to reduce your risk of developing these health conditions? The same applies to your loved ones— share what you learn freely or simply pass this book along. Together, we have the power to profoundly impact not only our own health but also the well-being of those around us.

Thank you for trusting me to be a part of your health journey. Now, let's get started.

Looking at Health Through the Lens of Inflammation

During my hospital rounds one warm July day, I got an urgent text from a nurse: "We need you in room 318 STAT!" I immediately dropped the consult I had been writing up and ran to the room, where I met Michelle, a transfer patient from a smaller local hospital.

Michelle had been suffering with ulcerative colitis for several years. Despite taking her prescribed medication religiously, she still had flare-ups of abdominal pain, bloody diarrhea, fatigue, and loss of appetite. Then about a week before I met her, she accidentally nicked herself shaving her legs. Two days later she developed a warm, red, tender, and very swollen leg. She went to urgent care and was prescribed Clindamycin, an antibiotic with good skin coverage, including for *Staph aureus*.

The antibiotics upset her stomach, and soon her bowels started to run loose, day and night. She figured this was just something that comes with the antibiotics, so she started using loperamide, a drug to slow bowel motility, around the clock. That way she could get some rest at night and work during the day.

Little did Michelle know that this wasn't just antibiotic-associated diarrhea. The Clindamycin had impacted her microbiome in a way that, by decimating the beneficial bacteria, had allowed a nasty pathogen called *Clostridioides difficile* to flourish. *C. diff* tears into the colon, leaving it raw, ulcerated, and a bloody mess. The body tries to flush out the bacteria with severe diarrhea, but when you take antidiarrheal medicine you actually trap it, allowing the pathogen to multiply and exponentially increase its inflammatory influence over the body. In just a few days, Michelle found herself being rushed to the emergency room with end-stage colon inflammation called toxic megacolon, so severe that surgical removal of the colon should be considered. When her body wasn't responding well to a maxed-out combination of oral and IV antibiotics, she was transferred to my hospital. By the time I met her she was delirious, unaware of where she was or what was going on. She had a high fever, a racing heart, and so much abdominal pain that if you accidentally bumped into her bed she would scream.

Most people would look at what happened with Michelle and see a severe infection. It seems so obvious. But I saw something different, a bigger picture that explained where her problem started. Michelle's health crisis began with the breakdown of the microscopic defense systems that protect her—a chain reaction starting with the decimation of her gut microbiome by antibiotics that were meant to help her. And everything that she experienced—high fever, racing heart, bloody and tattered intestines—was the consequence of severe inflammation, not a direct effect of the infection. Her symptoms were bodily manifestations of her immune system triggering a level five code red.

Surely you've heard this word—"inflammation"—tossed around. It's a bit buzzy. But what most don't realize is that inflammation occurs because your immune system is feeling threatened, and the science that has emerged in the past decade indicates that this chain reaction starts with the gut. We call it the gut-immune connection.

To really get to the root of inflammation, you need to zoom in on the microscopic parts of our body, where you'll find the gut microbes, the immune cells, and the paper-thin gut barrier that separates them. These three parts, each of which is invisible to the naked eye yet intricately linked with one another, form the foundation of our defense system and are the main determinants of inflammation in our body. New research has revealed that they are interconnected so powerfully that they will grow stronger or weaker *together*. This discovery opens up new opportunities for healing: We can heal the gut in order to heal the immune system.

The solution for Michelle to turn the corner, heal, and recover wasn't more antibiotics to destroy the pathogen. We were already maxed out on that approach, and she was getting worse. It may seem counterintuitive, but we flipped our strategy to healing her microbiome, which then naturally rebalanced her immune system and restored her defense systems—allowing her body to clear the infection on its own. This new paradigm—heal the gut to reduce inflammation and restore the immune system—is what I did for Michelle, and it's what we're here to do together in this book. The world is facing an epidemic of inflammatory diseases, and it's clear that our current approach isn't working. It's time to reimagine inflammation as a gut-driven process and focus our energy on healing from the inside out.

You don't have to have a health crisis as serious as Michelle's to be feeling the effects of inflammation that begins in the gut. Symptoms range from the less severe, like fatigue, bloating, and other digestive discomfort, joint pain, menopause symptoms, and feeling down or having brain fog to more serious conditions like autoimmune disease, endometriosis or PCOS (polycystic ovary syndrome), thyroid issues, and even cardiovascular disease and many cancers. During my two decades as a clinician, I began to notice that more and more of my patients who came in for their digestive issues would tell me they were also recently diagnosed with diabetes, cancer, long COVID, autoimmune diseases, and more. They were having heart attacks or being diagnosed with Alzheimer's disease. I couldn't ignore the feeling that there was a connection between these chronic diseases and the gut, so I decided to dive into the deep end of the pool. My gut instincts were on point—I found that there's a triangular connection between many diseases, gut health, and inflammation. It makes sense, actually. Seventy percent of the immune system lives in the gut. Both the immune system and your gut microbes call your gut home, and they are next-door neighbors. I know some people might tell me as a gastroenterologist to stay in my lane, but these gut origins are so powerful that this actually is my lane—gut-immune health.

If you have digestive issues, IBS (irritable bowel syndrome), ulcerative colitis, or even something as common as allergies that just seem to get worse every year, you are likely suffering from an inflammatory condition that begins in the gut. If you are experiencing a cascade of symptoms that may have started with digestive pain but now has grown to include chronic fatigue, stuffy nose, depressed mood, poor sleep, skin changes, and headaches, inflammation is most certainly a part of what's going on. If you have cancer, a heart condition, diabetes, obesity, or are struggling with menopause symptoms or to get an erection, yup, these are tied to inflammation, too. There is a very long list of things you don't think are related to your immune system but are—Parkinson's disease, arthritis, fatty liver disease, and fertility issues—and they all start in the gut.

This is not to claim that your gut microbiome is solely responsible for all inflammatory disease in the body, but it is to say that your gut microbes are so closely tied to your immune system that when the immune system is sick, the gut is as well. The gut is the gateway both to health and illness. And so it's even more important that if you're dealing with an inflammatory health condition, whether that be autoimmune, metabolic, cardiovascular, hormonal, or mood and brain health, that you intentionally nurture a healthier gut microbiome as a springboard to healing the immune system. That's how we got Michelle not only out of the ICU but feeling better than she had in years. The gut-immune connection is so powerful that by simply restoring her gut microbiome, we got Michelle up off her deathbed and walking out of the hospital in two days.

In Michelle's case, we made her gut healthy again by giving her a fecal transplant, a procedure in which fecal material from someone with a healthy microbiome is transferred to the gastrointestinal tract of a sick person, allowing the beneficial microbes from the donor to fight off the bad gut bugs and reestablish a balanced microbiome. But it's not enough to just pop a new engine under the hood. That engine needs fuel. The fecal transplant was just the beginning of a life transformation I helped her make with diet and lifestyle changes to power up her microbiome, to suppress the *C. diff* infection so it never came back, and to get her ulcerative colitis in such a deep remission that she lives her days not even thinking about it. That's next-level healing.

In 2020, my book *Fiber Fueled* took the world by storm by singing the praises of eating fiber-rich plant foods to tap into the healing energy that exists in the microbiome. But healing the gut microbiome is NOT one size fits all. Yes, there are foundational rules that apply to most, if not all, of us. But sometimes we need a more tailored strategy. Through the years, I've always wanted to provide that individualized approach to my patients with chronic inflammatory disorders like Crohn's disease and ulcerative colitis. But in truth, these methods extend far beyond those specific conditions because of the laundry list of health issues—our modern epidemics—that share a single root cause, a shared ancestor: chronic inflammation.

Conventional treatments for chronic inflammatory conditions often leave much to be desired. If you've picked up this book because you're one of the fifty million Americans suffering from a chronic autoimmune condition, you've likely tried lots of things to calm the cascade of inflammatory symptoms you experience. While most medical doctors rely on prescription medications and surgery to manage symptoms, health influencers and functional medicine folks often focus on elimination diets and detoxes that leave people with overly restrictive, nutritionally depleted diets—all in an attempt to prevent any kind of digestive response. Unfortunately, these extreme diets work in the short term, but they aren't sustainable. And what we *really* want is to be healthier in the long term. Following these kinds of diet fads can feel like you're riding the roller coaster, whiplashing from low carb to high carb, fruitarian to carnivore. Let me tell you something: The most popular diet may change every three years, but your biology doesn't change, and neither does the science. Trendy diets put marketing above real research.

If you've read my first book, you might be able to guess why I don't feel satisfied with either end of this spectrum. Medications and surgery are powerful tools, but they don't treat the underlying issue; they just manage your symptoms. Elimination diets are protocols for avoidance, but I have an added gripe with them: They take away your most precious resource for your health, the diversity of plant foods in your diet. In essence, while they claim to get to the "root cause" of your symptoms, they are still just another symptom management protocol. Elimination diets are probably healthier in some ways than taking loads of antibiotics, but they have their own health risks because they make the gut more fragile. The bottom line is that neither approach takes advantage of our greatest asset when it comes to the immune system: our microbiome.

If you've ever felt frustrated by the health advice you're given by doctors or the claims you read online, you are not alone. Not by a long shot. But here's the good news: Rock-solid science receives little hype, but slow and steady, it keeps charging forward. We know much more about the gut-immune connection today than when I wrote *Fiber Fueled* in 2019, and I'm excited to share this new understanding with you. We can use science to match your diet to your biology and achieve long-term anti-inflammatory health.

The research is clear that it is time for a paradigm shift: We should spend less time looking at the immune system and more time looking at the gut to address inflammation. If you want to stop the giant snowball rolling down the hill, it's a lot easier to control it when it fits in your hand rather than waiting until you're Indiana Jones and that snowball is ready to roll over you.

Here's the missing piece: The job of the microbiome is to train the immune system. The immune system is not just aimlessly floating around in our bodies; it needs to be—and can be—taught and educated by our gut microbes. We can make the most impact in the immune system by way of the microbiome.

In researching this book, I asked myself a simple question: How many of our most common, most recognizable health conditions are connected in some way to inflammation? What I discovered was jaw dropping. I found over 130 conditions connected to inflammation: from autoimmune, cardiovascular, hormonal, and metabolic conditions to cancers and neurological and psychiatric conditions. It's a very long, all-encompassing list. See for yourself on page 371. You could go to five different doctors for five different health conditions that are all tied together by one mechanism—inflammation. Yet you may never hear them say the word "inflammation" because each individual physician has been trained for years to identify the diagnosis in which they specialize and then prescribe something to help it. The result is that you end up on multiple medicines to reduce symptoms, but you never really get to the root. We break medicine into separate fields of study, but that's not the way that the body works. We have to see the whole picture if we want to truly heal.

When we can see our health from this holistic perspective rather than as clusters of symptoms and disconnected diagnoses, we can see that inflammation is trying to tell us something. It's telling us that the immune system is confused, threatened, and as a result not doing its job well. These characteristics are what show up when the immune system is disconnected and deprived of its intended healthy, collaborative relationship with the gut microbiome. There's a lot we can do to improve your microbiome, restore its ability to support the immune cells, and accomplish our end goal, which is a healthy, thriving immune system with less inflammation. The diet and lifestyle choices I explain in this book will trigger chain reactions through your body so that a cascade of healing ensues. The interconnected nature of our biology means that when we heal the gut, we reduce inflammation and undermine the diseases that are stuck in that gut-immune triangle.

This book was inspired by my patients with Crohn's disease and ulcerative colitis. I felt they deserved a solution beyond lifelong medication that often has nasty side effects, or a hyper-restrictive diet that's 50 percent red meat and eliminates whole categories of fiber-rich foods. As I worked to solve this problem, it became clear that we ALL benefit from an anti-inflammatory, gut-nourishing approach. It is the ultimate road map for longevity.

I call it Plant Powered Plus. The goal of the program is to create a foundation of health in your body through plant-based foods that feed and fuel a healthier gut microbiome. This is how we tame the flames of inflammation. But the "Plus" means there's more, much more. We will create consistency and use light exposure to foster biological rhythm around mealtimes, fasting, sleep, and supplement use. We will reconnect with ourselves, with others, and with our higher power to foster better emotional and spiritual health. We're going to talk about trauma, and that may be the key to unlocking better health for some of you.

While our foundation is plant-based food, my goal is to meet you where you are and to help you tailor your choices for your individual needs. People from all dietary backgrounds and perspectives are welcome here. Some of you are new to this, as I once was, and I want to give you space to grow. Some of you have serious health issues that you're battling, and you need to include some animal-based foods in order to fulfill your nutritional needs. And some of you simply prefer or feel better with the inclusion of some animal-based foods. I accept all of this as part of our process together and I will help guide you toward healthier choices along the way. I want to match you to an anti-inflammatory diet that fits your biology and your current medical needs and that is sustainable. It should be a way of eating that you can enjoy and adapt through the years.

None of the guidance in this book is predetermined or agenda driven. My only motive is your health, and our path is guided by a scientific compass. Every piece of advice is anchored in rigorous science. We're going to ultimately get to our goal, but the path to get there will be your own. If you're familiar with my first two books, you'll see some common elements, such as a plant-forward, plant-centered focus. But more than that, this approach highlights what you can add to your life to power your health, not what you need to take away. I want you thriving through abundance rather than suffering through deprivation.

In Part I of this book, I'll show you the very cool—and surprising—science behind how the immune system and the gut work together. Spoiler alert: This ancient relationship started long before humans even existed, although we have invented some very interesting ways to wreak havoc on it. Then we'll look at how inflammation is the root of autoimmune and other chronic immune conditions, how it emerges when the gut-immune relationship breaks down, and why plants offer the most powerful path to restoring this essential connection. We'll also address any lingering fears you may have about plant foods—especially if you've been told to eliminate them to keep your symptoms at bay—and explore how reintroducing them may actually support your healing journey.

In Part II, we'll explore how to heal your gut through nutrition, identify the pillars of an anti-inflammatory diet, create a circadian rhythm, fasting, and exercise timing—plus we'll learn practical tips for better sleep and a full breakdown on which supplements to take and *when* to take them. We'll finish by exploring the brain-gut-immune connection, revealing how our mind and soul impact the body and profoundly shape our overall health.

Finally in Part III, I'll put it all together for you in a protocol that is right for you with recipes and targeted, staged interventions to get you well on your way to a more harmonious gut-immune system relationship. This isn't a "three weeks to health" plan—it's a gradual, sustainable process. The time it takes to heal is highly individual. That's why this protocol is designed to meet you where you are, adapt to your needs today, and grow with you over time. Ultimately, you'll be embracing an anti-inflammatory diet and lifestyle—one that helps you feel better now and also propels your health forward for years to come.

You may already know me, but in the event that you don't, let's back up. Hi, I'm Dr. B. My lifelong dream was to be a physician and make a positive impact in the lives of others. Now I build tools for healing, including this book. I wake up every day excited by the possibility that you—yes, YOU—might find me and allow me to make a difference in your life. Recently, a woman stopped me in LaGuardia Airport, tears rolling down her face, to tell me that my work had changed her life. I can't tell you how much moments like that mean to me. My readers, including you, continue to inspire me.

To get to where I am today, I've been what you might call a grinder. I've spent most of my life clocking early mornings, late nights, weekends, and holidays. I still do, actually, but I'm working on it. (Let me know if you have any good book recs.) I've repeatedly been called an overachiever, which used to hurt my feelings but is now a cherished part of my self-identity. I have a bachelor's degree from Vanderbilt (in chemistry), a master's degree from Northwestern (in clinical investigation), and a medical degree from Georgetown. I trained at top hospitals with renowned doctors and won the highest award they gave every time. Through the years I've done my fair share of research. I earned a competitive award from the National Institutes of Health, and my research has been published in *Nature Medicine, Gastroenterology, Gut Microbes,* and many more. My work has been cited more than five thousand times by other researchers, an honor that reflects genuine respect in our field and fuels my drive to keep expanding the boundaries of what we know.

But above all, I'm a clinician at heart. It's my passion, why I went into medicine, and what I do best. While others may specialize in statistics, research methods, or rat studies, my expertise is in treating patients—real people with real health issues. I've always thrived caring for patients with the biggest challenges. I enjoy peeling back the layers of complexity and creating individualized plans for healing. I'm driven by results and committed to helping people achieve them—no polarizing groupthink will stand in the way. As a kid, I saw these divisions in politics and religion, but now this same divisive thinking has taken over nutrition, and it's holding us back. Your diet is NOT your identity, there is no shame in food, and it doesn't matter what other people think because this is about YOU. Different people thrive on different diets. Instead of forcing you into a rigid one-size-fits-all box, I want to help you break free from dogma and seek truth—rooted in science, applied in a way that works for your life, and designed to help you thrive. It's time to start over fresh and focused. That's my goal with my Plant Powered Plus plan.

No matter who you are, I want you to know that I see you and it is my mission to empower you. Let's go!

The Introduction is backed by 45 references gathered through an extensive review of the scientific literature. You can browse the full citation list at www.theguthealthmd.com/plantpoweredplus.

PART I

FOUNDATIONS OF INFLAMMATION

How Evolution and Environment
Shape the Gut-Immune Axis

CHAPTER 1

DEEP TIES
The Gut-Immune Connection

Starting in early 2020, discussions about immunity leapt into the global spotlight like never before. We've all witnessed a barrage of news segments and social media posts on handwashing, germ killing, stopping the spread of disease, immune system weakening, and inflammation, not just from COVID but also things like measles and *Listeria* outbreaks. And while this certainly has been an unprecedented time, those of us working in the medical field have long had the issue of immunity on our minds as we've seen patient after patient fight their immune system, a protective network that is supposed to defend them but for some reason commits bodily treason and attacks them. This attack could present as an autoimmune or allergic disease or chronic inflammation—all of these issues are exploding. Between 1970 and 2010, new Crohn's disease and ulcerative colitis cases increased by 55 percent and 33 percent in Olmsted County, Minnesota, where they closely track these things. This is not just in the United States. Between 1985 and 2015, new cases of autoimmune diseases increased by a staggering 19.1 percent *per year* across the globe. Nearly one in three adults now have seasonal allergies, eczema, or a food allergy.

The pandemic brought our attention to the immune system, but we probably should have been paying attention already because our problems actually started decades ago. The reality is that we're facing an epidemic that was fully underway before the COVID-19 coronavirus came around in the first place. There's a new wave of diseases that include autoimmune, allergic, and chronic inflammatory conditions that really started in the mid-twentieth century. They're here, and I'd argue that they're much more of a threat to us than the pandemic ever was.

The solution is not going to be one simple thing. The wellness industry sells you "immune-boosting" herbs, beverages, and diets, and frankly they're a crock of you-know-what. Sorry, but loading up on vitamin C isn't going to fix your problems and true healing is not going to come from single nutrients. Similarly, I've spent more than a decade celebrating the role our gut microbes play in our health. I'm a huge believer. But while our gut microbes are going to play an essential role in this story, it's not just about them.

To properly tell the story of gut-immune health, we have to shine a light on the legendary triad of bodily defenders—your gut microbes, gut barrier, and immune system—that serve as the heroes of your health. If this were a superhero movie, they would be working together as a powerhouse team to keep you healthy and safe. The collective whole is greater than the individual parts because they complement one another so well. But every good superhero movie is defined by having a formidable villain, the existential threat to our existence. In this story, that is lipopolysaccharide, which is the Voldemort or Darth Vader of gut health. Can you hear the ominous music as our villain makes its menacing entrance? You'll hear it in Chapter 2. But spoiler alert: Following the Plant Powered Plus Protocol in Chapter 9 will flip the script and set you on a path to triumphant gut-immune health. Before we jump into the conflict, let's begin at ground zero for all things gut health—your intestines.

A River Runs Through You

Your gut is where the outside world most powerfully interacts with your inner world—arguably the single most important interface for your long-term health. Yes, your skin and lungs do meet the external environment, but more in a protective or air-filtering capacity. In the gut, however, three to five pounds of food pass through daily—that's between one and two thousand pounds a year—every morsel completely foreign to your body.

Eating is, at its core, an act of trust. You could have spit it out, but you didn't—you're inviting it into some of your most vulnerable spaces. Let's pretend for a moment that we're on a high-stakes water slide tour through your intestines. After being chewed and knocked around by surging waves of saliva (we're off to a lovely start), you get briskly plunged down a dark tunnel that opens like a trapdoor (you just got swallowed), passing quickly through the esophagus before splashing into the stomach. There you get mixed and swirled around for a period of time in an acid bath (sorry about that) before circling the drain and plunging down into the small intestine. We call it small because the tube is tight, but it's really friggin' long, about twenty feet. By comparison, the large intestine, which is also called the colon, is just five feet long. It's short but notably broader.

Ideally, the intestines are like a river that brings fresh water and life-giving nutrients to your body. But often they also carry potentially perilous invaders or noxious substances. When the river is healthy, the surrounding lands benefit from the resources that it provides. Digestion is the process in which your body identifies those life-giving nutrients, separates them from everything else in the river, and pulls them into the body for your benefit. When this process is working perfectly, your intestines stay completely separate from the rest of your body, and an impenetrable barrier between the two allows only the good stuff to cross over. But it's very easy for this magical system to go awry. We consume well north of a million milligrams of food each day, some of which will be just what our body needs and some of which will disrupt our physiology. It puts a lot of stress on our body not to make a mistake.

When your food takes its journey through the intestines, it is just millimeters away from your bloodstream. If it gets in your blood, it can reach your brain or any of your other vital organs in a matter of seconds. It makes sense that the body would want to keep intestinal contents contained and separate. For one, it's poop; I'm pretty sure you don't want that mixing with your blood. But more specifically, poop contains some dangerous microbes that would love to enter your bloodstream and raise hell, like *E. coli* or *Pseudomonas*. Don't get me wrong, there's plenty inside the intestinal tube that is good for you. Depending on what you've chosen to eat, it may contain valuable resources that are required to maintain bodily functions. But it may also be filled with those microbes that are toxic and harmful to the body. That's why it's better to keep things separate until your body can vet the contents of your intestines and be sure it is safe.

The surface of the intestine measures about thirty-two square meters. That's roughly the size of a small studio apartment or two parking spaces side by side. It's a remarkable amount of surface area. But more importantly, every speck of that space has its own community of microbes, providing more opportunity for nutrients to be absorbed, but also more chances for invaders to slip in if defenses falter.

We should have the strongest defenses in the most vulnerable areas of our body. And we do. Thankfully, you have been blessed with a trio of bona fide superheroes standing guard at the gates: your gut microbes, your gut barrier, and your immune system. Any would-be intruder aiming to breach your body needs to get past all three. We can't afford to have them weak, tired, and confused. Using the information in this book, we're going to have them shields raised, fired up, and ready to defend you.

Your First Line of Defense: Your Microbes

A force of nature lives inside of you. You may remember them from my first book—they're those thirty-eight trillion microorganisms that are not human, nor are they a part of you. They're your gut microbes. We call them *micro* because they are invisible to the naked eye. Thank goodness, because they're literally floating over the top of your eyeball as you read this, and trying to read a good book through a swarm of microbes would be a total nightmare. But make no mistake, they're there.

Let's pull a microscope out for a moment and take a look together. Most of these microorganisms exist in your colon. As we peer down into the recesses of your bowels, what you see are mostly bacteria. These are free-living organisms that each consist of just one biological cell. That doesn't sound like much, but when you consider that there are thirty-eight trillion of them and you have just thirty trillion human cells, you are clearly, irrefutably less than half human. You're outnumbered!

These organisms are not just bacteria. There are also billions of fungi, which are more complicated in that they contain a cellular structure more closely resembling humans. There may also be archaea and protozoa. Archaea are somewhere between bacteria and fungi, and we believe they're the oldest life on the planet. Archaea are known for producing methane gas. Scientists have found evidence of archaea burping methane gas near hydrothermal vents 3.4 billion years ago, and now they burp methane gas within your colon. It's a family tradition! Meanwhile, scientists are also discovering that protozoa, which can include creepy worms and parasites, are in some cases beneficial to our health. More on that later.

Much like us, these microbes are diverse. There are typically five hundred to a thousand species of bacteria and fifty to one hundred species of fungi in your body at any one time. Different microbes do different things. Each microbe has different skills that contribute to the collective whole, where the sum of the microbes is capable of far more than the individual contributions. They exist in communities and tend to seek out like-minded friends to support one another. They have different temperaments. Some of them are sweet and friendly. These are the beneficial bacteria, like *Lactobacillus* and *Bifidobacterium*. Others are downright nasty. We call these pathogens, like the *C. diff* from the Introduction, or *E. coli* or *Salmonella*. Every day the whole community of microbes wakes up and adapts to their environment, seeking out safety and sustenance, with hopes to make babies and enjoy a delicious meal. Does their world sound a bit like your world? That's because they exist in a parallel metaverse. Theirs is microscopic; yours is macroscopic. But they exist in this microscopic microcosm of *your* life. We have officially entered the matrix.

Don't get too full of yourself, but you are a god to them. Not figuratively. Literally. You have the ability to create violent storms and earthquakes, to change when the sun goes up and comes down, to select the fortunate winners and the unfortunate losers. That's because your choices influence their environment, and ultimately they are the product of that environment. Families of microbes rise and fall based upon the conditions.

The choices you make have a rapid, massive impact on them. If you change your diet, you will change your microbiome. In fact, it will happen very quickly. Within twenty-four hours of food hitting your colon, your microbiome will be different, shaped by the food that passed through. Rapid changes in the microbiome are facilitated by rapid microbial turnover. A single microbe could spawn over a thousand offspring in a single day. Think about that. It's an incredible superpower.

The conditions in your colon, their environment, matter. It's not just what you eat that matters. When you eat and how you eat matters, too. As do non-dietary factors like sleep, exercise, stress, and human connection. They all contribute to the context that shapes your microbiome. We'll be taking a deep dive into all of this in Part II of this book, and it is SUPER cool.

When most people think of the gut, digestion springs to mind. That's true—our microbes break down food and even medications. But these microbes do much more than convert calories into energy. They function like a bustling chemical factory, synthesizing a vast array of bioactive compounds that ripple throughout the body, influencing metabolism, hormones, mood, and cognition. Their most critical impact, however, lies mere micrometers away, where they directly interact with the gut barrier and immune cells. In this microscopic zone, gut microbes are pivotal in regulating inflammation, training immune responses, and ultimately guiding how well your entire immune system defends you.

Your Second Line of Defense: Your Gut Barrier

Flowing through your intestines are substances you absolutely want your body to absorb—like nutrients and vitamins. Meanwhile, your microbes do a remarkable job of breaking down and transforming many of the compounds that pass through. But they can't do it all by themselves and they're not really designed to separate and compartmentalize. Walls are built for a reason. You need a selective filter that allows the good stuff in while keeping harmful substances locked in the tube, destined for elimination. Where microbes leave off, superhero #2 takes over—give it up for the gut barrier.

Your gut barrier is a single layer of cells, also known as the epithelium, that acts as a filter between your bloodstream and your gut bacteria. On top of this layer of cells is a layer of mucus, which adds extra protection to the gut barrier. This slimy, gelatinous substance serves many purposes—lubrication, protection from invasive bacteria, and even a home and nutrient source for some friendly bacteria. Embedded in the mucus layer you'll find all kinds of defensive substances—antimicrobial proteins, immunoglobulins, and enzymes—that help keep the invasive bacteria out. With a microscope, you can literally measure the thickness of the juicy mucus layer. We want it to be not just thick but thicky thick. A thin mucus layer means less protection and increased exposure to infection as well as a greater risk of colon cancer, ulcerative colitis, type 2 diabetes, obesity, and nonalcoholic fatty liver disease. The good news is that our food choices exert some control over the thickness of the mucus layer. More on that soon.

Together, the gut barrier and the mucus layer are like a wall and moat separating the untamed wilderness from the manicured garden within. This biological firewall needs to strike a delicate balance: If it's too weak, unwanted invaders slip through; if it's too tough, essential nutrients get shut out. The cells in the gut barrier serve as the bricks in a wall. The bricks are held together by special proteins called tight junctions, nature's cement. Tight junctions fasten the cells together, keeping the harmful pathogens out while allowing water and electrolytes to pass. But if they break down, we lose control. The gut barrier is no longer intact. The invasive microbes and toxins will find the weakness, like rats finding the smallest hole in your house. They'll wiggle their way between the cells, through the wall, and once they're across it's a mad dash into the bloodstream.

The gut barrier isn't just a wall. It's an immune organ. In fact, it's the dominant immune organ in your body. Barrier breaches can happen at any moment, anywhere within the intricate thirty-two-square-meter landscape that is your gut. Remember how I said every speck matters? Now I'm emphasizing that every microscopic fraction of that speck matters. Your gut barrier is the one thing present across the entire surface area to protect you, and every cell and every tight junction matters. And now you know why 70 percent of your immune system lies in the gut. It's that important.

What happens if the bad guys sneak past the gut microbes, through the mucus layer, and past a hole in the gut barrier? They may be feeling pretty good about themselves, until they look up and see our final hero towering over them: the immune system.

Your Third Line of Defense: Your Immune System

Your immune system's complexity is limitless—we could get lost for an eternity trying to understand all of it. I'm going to do my best to keep it relatively simple, but know that if you want to be an immunologist one day, there's an entire network of rabbit holes out there for you to explore.

Let's take it from the top: The immune system is a network of organs, cells, and proteins whose purpose is to protect you and your tissues. That includes neutralizing pathogens and squashing infections. If a pathogen dares to invade, it must first get past the gut's resident microbial defenders (our first hero), slip through the mucus layer, and breach the gut barrier (our second hero). And if, by some miracle, it survives all that, a vigilant squad of innate immune cells on the other side stands ready to fend off invaders until the supercharged adaptive immune cells arrive and—BOOM—it's game over. It also means damage control and repair when there's bodily injury. To accomplish all of this, we have two bureaus of defense—the innate immune system and the adaptive immune system. Let's explore them.

The Innate Immune System: For Fast, Everyday Protection

The innate immune system is our workhorse, designed to handle most things that require activation of our immune system from day to day.

It is pretrained, which allows it to immediately respond to any threat. No learning necessary! This allows it to be fast, but you sacrifice strength and effectiveness for speed. That's okay, though, because for most mundane tasks, the innate immune system is just fine.

We tend to think of the immune system as being cells, but it's much more. The innate immune system starts with physical barriers, like the skin or the gut barrier, both of which separate the outside from the inside. Then there are the chemical substances that neutralize pathogens, like the mucus layer, which contains protective substances to keep invasive bacteria out. Other examples include oil on your skin, tears from your eyes, saliva in your mouth, and acid in your stomach. All of these are antimicrobial, designed to eliminate or keep our microbes from getting into the body.

The innate immune system also includes cells called white blood cells, or leukocytes. There are several unique types—macrophages, neutrophils, natural killer cells, and others—each with slightly different strengths or functions that contribute to the overall goal of protecting you.

Immune cells operate independent of your brain and consciousness, but let's not make them sound too smart. They're more like robots that are preprogrammed to react in specific ways to specific situations. Don't get me wrong: The innate immune system is insanely intelligent. Thousands of scientists have devoted their lives to understanding it and they still haven't figured it all out, but its capabilities are very different from the human brain. Instead, the intelligence of your innate immune system is the glorious result of millions (if not billions) of years of evolution. What worked got carried forward.

Your white blood cells have the ability to get organized and work in teams to take on a threat. This requires cellular communication and coordination, which is possible thanks to messenger proteins that we call cytokines. Envision your immune cells as a tactical team on a mission, each equipped with a walkie-talkie (i.e., cytokines) to call for backup or share intel. They act as a form of communication among immune cells, allowing them to organize and coordinate their behavior. Perhaps you've heard of some of these—interleukin-1 (IL-1), IL-6, IL-17, tumor necrosis factor alpha (TNFα), and interferon gamma (IFNγ). These are examples of cytokines that are known to fire up the immune system and send it to war. In fact, we treat various inflammatory diseases like ulcerative colitis, rheumatoid arthritis, psoriasis, and even COVID-19 with FDA-approved drugs designed to block these cytokines—they're that central to your immune system response. The immune cells are the soldiers and the cytokines are their marching orders—activate for war, or chill in the barracks.

The Adaptive Immune System: When You Need Targeted Support

The innate immune system is great for most rudimentary tasks, but sometimes the body needs the immune system to be more targeted. This is why we have the adaptive immune system, which is made up of special white blood cells called lymphocytes. They're like the special forces of the immune system. They're more complex, more precise, and far more powerful. They are biological badasses that are not to be messed with. The lymphocytes step up when the innate immune system struggles to get the job done. In comes the heavy artillery, as the lymphocytes pull out weapons of war called antibodies that function like precision-guided missiles.

When lymphocytes encounter something for the first time (as happened during the pandemic with the coronavirus), you have to give them four or five days to build out their munitions. But once the antibodies are developed, they can be rapidly deployed at any time in the future. The second encounter with a pathogen will be more rapid and effective than the first. This is what we call immune memory, and it

13

allows your immune system to grow stronger with each encounter—ensuring faster, more effective responses in the future.

Your Microbes, Gut Barrier, and Immune System Rise and Fall Together

Your immune system and your gut are deeply interconnected and inseparable. When your gut is balanced and teeming with healthy microbes, it helps repair and restore your gut barrier and train and regulate your immune system so that it's primed to respond appropriately to real threats. From birth, our gut microbiome "educates" our immune system by exposing it to a diverse range of microbes. This helps immune cells learn what's normal and what's a threat, reducing the risk of overreactions—like allergies or autoimmune diseases. Our gut microbes produce bioactive chemicals—neurotransmitters, bile acid and tryptophan metabolites, and, most importantly, short-chain fatty acids—that interact with and manipulate the immune system. And last but not least, the good gut microbes play an important role in maintaining the gut barrier, which protects the immune system and allows it to do its job more effectively. But if these protective microbes are wiped out, the gut barrier starts to break down and your immune system can go haywire, and the entire defense system becomes weak, toothless, and more dangerous to you than your enemies.

Remember Michelle? She took a round of antibiotics for a skin infection and ended up with a vicious, life-threatening case of *C. diff* colitis. What was going on there? How did she end up with a raging immune system taking over her body and putting her on death's doorstep? And why did a fecal transplant, of all things, heal her?

It started with the injury to her gut microbes. Within days of starting the antibiotics, Michelle experienced a precipitous fall in the number of living bacteria and the diversity within her microbiome. I'm sure you've heard many of these terms—antibiotic, antimicrobial, antibacterial, germicide, bactericide. These are all variations on the same thing for gut bacteria: death. But you're not just killing the bad ones. Many of the bacteria lost are anti-inflammatory, like *Faecalibacterium prausnitzii*, which are critical to keeping the gut barrier intact. Meanwhile, the ones that survive are, by definition, antibiotic resistant. We call this dysbiosis, when the microbiome has fallen out of balance due to a loss of overall diversity, with fewer good ones and too many inflammatory bad ones. Dysbiosis affects the ability of the gut microbiome to do its job. In this case, the microbes lose their ability to repair and restore the gut barrier.

A damaged gut barrier—commonly called "leaky gut"—lets toxins slip across and come into direct contact with the immune system. Sensing a threat, the immune system releases inflammatory cytokines, which recruit more immune cells that also produce inflammatory cytokines, and the snowball of inflammation gets set in motion. What started as damage to the gut microbiome has now disrupted the gut barrier and set off the immune system, and the result is massive amounts of inflammation that makes the body very, very sick.

All it takes is a round of antibiotics and next thing you know, the microbes, gut barrier, and immune system are all dysfunctional and you have an inflammatory mess. Sounds like a delicate and vulnerable system, but it doesn't have to be. We can use the interconnectedness to our advantage, fighting inflammation by fortifying our gut microbes. Once healthy, these microbes will repair and restore the gut barrier for us, which protects the immune system and allows it to be strong.

Michelle's story exemplifies this. The antibiotics that triggered her health crisis weren't going to resolve it, so a fecal transplant from a healthy donor was the best option to increase her gut diversity quickly. Fecal transplants restore the beneficial gut microbes that suppress the

C. diff infection, rebuild the gut barrier, and reduce the passage of harmful toxins. In just a couple of days after her transplant, Michelle was already back on her feet, high-fiving me on her way out of the hospital.

Now, here's the good news for the rest of us. In most cases, you won't need a fecal transplant to heal your gut. And no, this book isn't about giving yourself a poop transplant. If it were, I would've called it *Poop Powered* (maybe next time?). The real key is harnessing the profound, interconnected relationship between the gut and the immune system.

The Key to a Healthy Gut and Immune Relationship Is . . .

Now we get to the important part: the one thing, the most important thing, that explains the interconnectedness of the microbes, gut barrier, and immune system. Are you ready for it? The answer is short-chain fatty acids.

In *Fiber Fueled* I introduced readers to these amazing molecules, of which there are three main types: acetate, made up of two carbon atoms; propionate, made of three; and butyrate, made of four. Friendly bacteria in our guts transform fiber into short-chain fatty acids, or SCFAs, which then work their magic by making your microbiome healthier. In my first book I talked about how SCFAs are anti-inflammatory, but now I'm doubling down: I've been studying science and medicine since 1998, and short-chain fatty acids are hands down *the* most anti-inflammatory thing that I've ever come across. Let's dive in.

SCFAs are produced by our anti-inflammatory gut microbes, like the *Faecalibacterium prausnitzii* that I mentioned above. Their healing effects start immediately and locally, right there in the gut. You get more beneficial bacteria like *Bifidobacteria*, *Lactobacilli*, and *Prevotella* that can help you produce more SCFAs. I showed you a snowball effect that creates inflammation. This is your anti-inflammatory snowball, which sets off a chain reaction that multiplies the anti-inflammatory microbes. Simultaneously, the SCFAs suppress inflammatory bacteria like *Salmonella*, *Shigella*, and *E. coli*. When you have more beneficial microbes and fewer inflammatory ones, your gut microbiome becomes balanced and lets the good guys take control. Nature is healing. This is how we fix dysbiosis.

A healthy gut microbiome produces the SCFAs that heal your gut barrier. Consider this: The intestinal epithelium sheds and replaces itself once every three to five days, which is the fastest rate of cellular turnover in the body. That, by itself, is quite marvelous. But even more interesting and exciting is the way in which we can shape and enhance all aspects of the new barrier with butyrate. Butyrate helps the body produce and introduce new, healthy cells through stem cell differentiation. As those new cells insert themselves like another brick in the wall, butyrate helps create the proteins that form the tight junctions. This acts like the cement—it holds it together and makes the wall impenetrable. With the wall now intact, butyrate activates goblet cells (microscopic slime cannons) to produce more mucus, thickening up the mucus layer that forms the outer protective layer.

Basically, what I'm telling you is that all of the steps to create a secure gut barrier, including a thick mucus layer, involve butyrate. And this is why, when the gut is dysbiotic and not producing enough butyrate, it thins the mucus layer in our colon; compromises the gut barrier, which becomes permeable; and ultimately allows invasion by pathogenic bacteria that promote inflammation.

When the gut barrier is secure, it prevents toxins from sneaking across and triggering your immune system. This drops levels of inflammatory cytokines such as NF-κB, TNF-α, IL-6, IL-1β, and IL-8—precisely the targets of many anti-inflammatory drugs, like infliximab and adalimumab. Simultaneously, butyrate promotes the release of IL-10, a cytokine shown to protect against inflammatory bowel disease.

In essence, the balance has shifted from inflammatory to anti-inflammatory when this happens.

> ### Should We Be Measuring SCFA Levels in Stool?
> Unfortunately, it's not reliable to measure SCFA levels in our stool. Butyrate provides 70 percent of the energy to power up your gut barrier, and anything not used for energy ends up getting absorbed. Just 5 percent of SCFAs end up in your poop. This is why measuring poop levels of SCFAs isn't extremely helpful, because it doesn't give an accurate picture of what's happening at the gut barrier or in the body.

Your body is starving for SCFAs, so anything not used by the gut barrier will get absorbed into the body, where it will float around without doing much until it comes into contact with a receptor. Receptors are the lock, and the SCFAs are the key. They fit together perfectly, and because they do, they are able to make things happen when they come together. As of this writing, we've identified six receptors for SCFAs, and what's fascinating is that four out of the six directly affect the immune system and inflammation. You'll find these receptors throughout the body, in the bone marrow and lymph nodes, and on the immune cells themselves.

One of the ways SCFAs influence your immune system is by shaping the innate immune system. In some ways, SCFAs are pumping the brakes. They do this throughout the body, even the bone marrow, slowing down the expansion and aggression of the immune system. For example, butyrate and propionate have been shown to reduce the production of inflammatory cytokines by monocytes. When you're pumping the brakes on the immune system and cooling down the immune cells, we have another word for it—anti-inflammatory.

In other ways, SCFAs help get the right cells on the battlefield. Think of them as generals, assessing the combat needs, calling up the right combination of soldiers, and putting them in the proper position to work together and eliminate a threat. Without battlefield leadership, you have chaos—too many of the soldiers you don't need, too few of the soldiers you do need, no one is talking to one another, and everyone is pointing the finger at the other. This is why we need SCFAs: to get the mission organized, to make it tactical and precise. It's what you want from your immune system, right? Thank you, SCFAs, for providing that.

But that's just the innate immune system. What about when we bring in the heavy weaponry—the T cells and the adaptive immune system? Once again, SCFAs have a general anti-inflammatory effect, pumping the brakes on the production and recruitment of T cells with one exception—T regulatory cells (Tregs). SCFAs actually stimulate the thymus to produce more T regulatory cells, such that in mice the concentration of SCFAs is proportional to the number of Tregs in the blood. T regulatory cells are like little peacekeepers because they are powerfully anti-inflammatory, they prevent autoimmunity, and they limit chronic inflammatory diseases. So we love that SCFAs give us more Tregs. Thank you, again, SCFAs, for providing that.

What if you have an infection, though? In these moments, you don't need immune suppression. But don't worry, because what SFCAs actually give you is an overall enhanced immune function. Butyrate helps the immune system properly recognize and remove invading microbes, thereby striking the proper balance of protecting you without creating unnecessary inflammation.

At this point you're wondering how we get more of that SCFA healing power, and the answer isn't a fecal transplant. It's something far simpler. Acetate, propionate, and butyrate are produced when prebiotic fiber (or resistant starch) comes into contact with the beneficial anti-inflammatory gut bugs. In fact, the reason why those gut bugs are anti-inflammatory is because they help you produce SCFAs. We'll dig more into the specifics of fiber in Chapter 5, but for right now what I want you to know is that short-chain fatty acids are powerfully anti-inflammatory because they connect the microbes to the gut barrier and immune system, and we get them from FIBER.

We Need Our Immune System Working for Us, Not Against Us

Your immune system isn't a simple on-off switch—it's an intricate, evolving dance that relies on both timely aggression and measured restraint. We need it to step up and do its job at the right times, and then other times we need it to calm down and stop picking fights. We want it to be precise. In order to do that, we need to protect the immune system, make it stronger, and empower it to do its job for us. We don't need to have it all figured out. Even our scientists don't have it all figured out. We just need to understand that there are literally billions of years of intelligence in our immune system. It's okay to trust that intelligence. And we need to be smart enough to see that it's the microbes that protect, strengthen, and empower the immune system. If you want to heal the immune system, you should heal the gut.

A perfectly functioning immune system will react only to those things that are harmful and will completely leave alone those that are not. Imprecise discrimination leads to inflammation that's violent, destructive, and totally unnecessary. Mistargeted inflammation in response to something foreign to the body—such as food proteins, pollen, or pet dander—is an allergic reaction. Errant and inappropriate inflammation in response to your own body is an autoimmune disorder—Hashimoto's, lupus, rheumatoid arthritis, multiple sclerosis, and many others. And wrongful inflammation in response to your gut microbiome causes inflammatory bowel diseases—Crohn's disease and ulcerative colitis. All of these are variations on a similar theme, which is the price we pay when our immune system is confused and attacking the wrong thing. But these are just *some* of the chronic inflammatory health conditions that pose an emerging threat in the last century. There is also a price to pay when the immune system is activated and creating chronic low-grade inflammation: Coronary artery disease, stroke, multiple forms of cancer, a wrecked metabolism with obesity and diabetes, fatty liver disease, hormonal issues, mood disorders, and dementia are just some of the medical issues that result. They are our modern epidemics.

An imprecise immune system can also fail to identify threats and fail in its job to protect us. It's not just infections. The body produces 3.8 million *new* human cells *every second*. Some of those cells are going to have mutations that make them cancerous. What that rate is depends on many factors such as genetics, environmental exposures, and inflammation. But even if we assume an insanely low rate, your body is still able to create cancer cells many times per day. It is the job of your immune system to identify and eliminate these abnormal cells. It's very, very good at this, thank goodness. But, there's zero margin for error. If a cancerous cell is able to evade the immune system, you know what eventually happens. This is why we need an immune system that precisely discriminates between friend and foe, benign and cancerous, beneficial and pathogenic.

Across the board, when we suppress the immune system, we increase our risk of infections and cancer. We see this in immunosuppressed conditions like acquired immunodeficiency syndrome (AIDS), where infections (pneumocystis pneumonia or tuberculosis) and cancer (non-Hodgkin lymphoma and Kaposi sarcoma) are the top threats.

Sometimes, when the immune system isn't pulling its weight, it needs to be pushed. Early in my career, I treated hepatitis C using interferon—a type of cytokine that revs up the immune system. In theory, this frenzy should wipe out the virus. But in practice, patients are forced to endure intense flu-like symptoms such as fever, chills, joint and muscle pains, headaches, and fatigue every time they inject themselves. Sadly, many patients would endure this for an entire year, only to find the virus still lingering. It was brutal. Thankfully, we have better ways to treat hepatitis C now.

More recently, cancer treatment has seen a breakthrough that refines this same idea: Rather than killing cancer cells directly with chemotherapy, we harness the body's own immune system by administering specific cytokines. We call this immunotherapy, and it's now being used to treat melanoma, breast cancer, non–small cell lung cancer, prostate cancer, and more. By empowering the immune system, immunotherapy can more precisely target the cancer cells while minimizing damage to healthy tissue, often resulting in greater efficacy that can lead to sustained responses to treatment. It's also customizable and therefore can be tailored to specific tumor types and in some cases individual patients' characteristics. Although immunotherapy often has side effects similar to interferon treatment—such as fatigue and flu-like symptoms—the targeted and precise manipulation of the immune system offers better results and longer-lasting cancer control. This is quickly changing the game in cancer.

But what if we could stop the cancer when it was just a single cell, way before it became a tumor? What if we could empower our immune system to function as precisely as possible, without needing to be suppressed or overactivated—and we could do it by simply changing our diet and lifestyle?

Your Microbiome Can Teach Your Immune System to Work Better

In *Fiber Fueled*, I told you that your gut is like a muscle. It can be trained. It can be made stronger. Challenges are good because they help you to level up your gut muscle. I'm here today to tell you that the same is true for your immune system. It is like a muscle. We are not born with the perfect immune system, but it can be trained and made stronger through challenges.

If the immune system is a muscle and it can be trained, then the next logical question is: Who is the teacher?

Your gut microbes, of course. They sit just micrometers away from 70 percent of your immune system. We aren't born with these microbes and they aren't human, nor are they a formal part of our body. Yet every single one of us acquires our gut microbiome at birth, and it is our invisible partner in life, evolving and adapting with us and for us. From start to finish, it works tirelessly to educate your immune system about what is good and what is bad.

In the gut, immune cells are perpetually exposed to microbes, food products, chemicals and contaminants, drugs, and whatever food was on your floor after you invoked the "10-second rule." It never stops. Every second of your existence, from the moment of your birth to your last day, with no breaks, your immune system stands as the sentinel protecting your body and attempting to understand what among this stuff is good and what is bad. That requires learning.

Let me show you how that learning works and how we can teach our immune system to do even better.

Chapter 1 is backed by 107 references gathered through an extensive review of the scientific literature. You can browse the full citation list at www .theguthealthmd.com/plantpoweredplus.

CHAPTER 2

EARLY ORIGINS
Understanding Root Causes and Our Evolutionary Past

One of the most perplexing aspects of the COVID-19 pandemic was the stark contrast in how individuals responded to the virus. Some people experienced few to no symptoms—perhaps they had a mild cough or a case of the sniffles, and they often didn't even realize they were carrying and potentially transmitting the virus. But others had a very different, much scarier, and potentially life-threatening experience. Their defenses collapsed, causing their organs to fail. They arrived at the hospital in desperate need of advanced life support just to give them a fighting chance. We call this septic shock—a life-threatening scenario caused by their immune system going into rage mode. When the immune system goes nuclear, it's really, really bad. But what's setting it off?

What you heard on the news during the height of COVID is that being older in age or having metabolic issues like diabetes or obesity put people at greater risk. But is it really just old age that makes people vulnerable to viruses? Or is there something more specific, a root cause that we can identify and address so that we're not sitting on our hands, waiting to be the victim of something we can't control?

The Destructive Power of LPS

What you weren't told is that in the first year of the pandemic we already knew that patients with severe COVID-19 had a large amount of something called lipopolysaccharide (LPS) coursing through their bloodstream. Further, those who died had higher LPS levels than those who survived. You could argue that these findings are merely associations and just markers of severe illness, but then researchers discovered that LPS actually binds to the COVID virus, forming a partnership that can intensify the disease. That discovery reveals a hidden synergy, redefining our understanding of how infection and inflammation work hand in hand.

But where does LPS come from in the first place—and how is it getting to the bloodstream? Lipopolysaccharide coats the outside of the pathogenic, inflammatory bacteria that live in your gut. We all have it, and that's a normal thing. Your good gut microbes and the short-chain fatty acids (SCFAs) they produce help to suppress those bad guys. When the body is in balance, the LPS gets compartmentalized to the intestines and there should be very little LPS in the bloodstream. But when the gut barrier is failing, LPS is able to sneak across, where it meets the immune system. Your immune system is programmed to identify and destroy LPS. Some LPS in your bloodstream is like a small leak in a boat—your immune system can easily bail out the water and keep things afloat. But when the gut barrier is severely compromised, it's like a gaping hole in the hull, flooding the boat faster than the immune system can handle, leading to widespread inflammation and immune dysfunction. That's when it's really easy for the immune system to overshoot: It goes full force in your defense, but it actually makes you sicker in the process.

Researchers found if mice had COVID without LPS, their infection was mild with little inflammation, perhaps like humans experiencing minor symptoms such as a stuffy nose or mild cough. If mice had high LPS but no COVID, the response was much stronger and more dangerous, causing systemic inflammation, akin to when humans experience body aches, brain fog, and extreme fatigue. This means LPS is a major driver of immune dysfunction. But when LPS combines with an infection, it unleashes a storm inside the body, pushing the immune system into rage mode. The outward signs of severe inflammation— high fever, widespread pain, gut distress, and overwhelming fatigue— are actually the result of something happening at a microscopic level—lipopolysaccharide combining with COVID to make the immune system go nuclear. Basically, what I'm telling you is that people aren't vulnerable to worse outcomes from COVID and other viruses because they're just "old." There's a powerful root cause at play, and LPS is a key part of the puzzle.

The issue for people who ultimately manifested severe COVID-19 was a weakened gut microbiome and a compromised gut barrier, leaving them vulnerable from the start. With both of these defenses down, LPS could slip into their bloodstream unchecked, forcing the immune system to step up and fight. This is how LPS creates a state of chronic low-grade inflammation. When the virus arrived, LPS was already in their system and their immune system was already embroiled in an inflammation battle, making it easier for LPS and COVID to join forces and ignite a massive inflammatory bomb in the body. I have the results of published studies to back me up. Here's what they reveal:

BROKEN BIOME

Those with an active COVID-19 infection showed more pathogenic, inflammatory microbes and fewer SCFA-producing ones.

BROKEN BARRIER

Severe COVID was associated with increased gut permeability.

BROKEN BIOME + BROKEN BARRIER = INFLAMMATION

The severity of inflammation and COVID infection correlated to the degree of dysbiosis and gut permeability.

On the flip side, those who followed a plant-based diet were less vulnerable to the effects of COVID. In fact, there are now multiple studies involving close to 650,000 people that collectively suggest that plant-based diets protect us from getting the infection, and if we get it we are less likely to have a severe case. In the last chapter, we discussed how the short-chain fatty acids we get from fiber (in plant-based foods) connect the gut microbiome to both the gut barrier and the immune system. In other words, they rise together.

I want you to see the interconnectedness that we're exposing here. In Chapter 1, I showed you that the gut biome, gut barrier, and immune system are in lockstep, rising and falling together. When they are collectively weak, toxins like LPS that naturally exist within our gut can cause harm and create low-grade inflammation, which has been associated with the myriad of diseases that I've listed on page 371. But this is more than just a microscopic war taking place inside your body. Something from the outside environment, such as a virus, could show up and the state of our biome, barrier, and immune system would determine the effects of that virus on our body. Simultaneously, what we ate for lunch and for dinner last night could provide the SCFAs that we need to improve the health of our biome, barrier, and immune system and bolster our resilience against that virus. This is just one example of how we are being shaped by our environment and our choices, which translates to our health in both the short term and the long term.

Everything in our environment, from the food we eat to the time of day and the relationships we have with others, contributes to these biome, barrier, and immune interactions. But in order to understand the whole picture and how to keep our defenses strong, we have to back up to look at how a chain of events spanning billions of years led to your existence and shaped how your body protects you.

The Ancient Origins of Our Immune System in Microbial Evolution

Let's travel back three billion years, when bacteria and archaea ruled Earth, creating the first ecosystems. Competition spurred the evolution of beneficial microbial characteristics that persist to this very day. First, these organisms developed bacteriocins that are like microbial spears. Our beneficial SCFA-producing bacteria use them to suppress inflammatory bacteria like *E. coli*, *Salmonella*, and even *C. difficile*. Interestingly, twenty-first-century scientists are now studying bacteriocins as "next generation" antibiotics, but I'm telling you that this has been a part of nature for billions of years already.

The inflammatory bacteria developed a form of microbial armor that protects them from bacteriocins and even antibiotics. This armor exists on the outside of the bacteria, like the plated scales of a prehistoric creature, providing a fierce protective edge and structural integrity. Over time, this molecular shield not only fortified the outer membrane of the inflammatory bacteria but also began to manage critical interactions with the environment, allowing these microbial survivors to thrive. This is the story of the evolution of LPS. Here comes the ominous soundtrack in the movie version of our history.

The development of LPS created connections between humans, microbes, and our immune system that are foundational to our physiology and ultimately our approach in this book. I mentioned that inflammation is what happens when your immune system feels threatened. LPS evolved to be the indicator of a threat. Your immune system has been programmed to identify and destroy anything that has LPS attached to it. In the beginning of the chapter I showed you the role that LPS plays in severe COVID. I'll come back to that in a minute.

Our species, *Homo sapiens*, first appeared about 150,000 years ago. Pretty recent compared to the 4-billion-year history of microbes. But I would argue that our human immune system started developing around 1.5 billion years ago. That's when single cells started to smash and pack together to form multicellular organisms for the first time. Suddenly, instead of a bazillion separate specks of dirt, we now had clay that could mold into stuff. What would you create? If you were making an animal you would give it legs to move, eyes to see, a nose to smell, and a hand to reach. These are major advantages to help find food and survive. But animals still need food, and the earth's soil holds nutrients that we'd like to transfer to those animals, so we create plants that have roots to harvest nutrients and leaves to capture energy from the sun. The plants are now the vehicle to transfer earth's nutrients and the sun's energy to the animals.

Multicellular life was an incredible opportunity for the single-celled microbes. It created new ecosystems that are less harsh, are less volatile, and provide a consistent source of nutrients. We may not think of body parts as ecosystems, but the skin, mouth, or intestine of an animal serves as home for a community of microbes. Imagine being a pioneering bacteria that discovers the inside of a mammalian intestine for the first time. You'd think:

*It's temperature controlled, food is being served all day—
all you can eat!—and at night it's quiet and safe.*

As life evolved and became more complex, more multicellular, one thing remained true. No matter what you created, it had a microbiome. It evolved with a microbiome. It was powered by its microbiome. That is universal. Whether it is an animal, a plant, a human, or something else, all multicellular life on this planet has a microbiome. There was no such thing as "sterile" in nature. Sterile is the result of humans creating unnatural conditions with their industrial chemicals. But in nature, microbes are ubiquitous. They're everywhere.

That means a committed partnership between multicellular and single-cellular life from day one. Every single second of every day for over a billion years has been a story of microbes and more complex life coexisting and thriving *together*. They made a pact with one another. Survival was mutually beneficial.

We are better with our microbes as our partners in life. But make no mistake, there's some risk involved. There are some microbes in there, the ones wearing a coat of LPS armor, that would love to raise hell if they could. When the good-guy microbes are strong, they use their bacteriocins to suppress the troublemakers, but in moments of weakness our good microbes may get overwhelmed. The result is an infection. This is why we evolved our immune system.

Our immune system didn't start with the first humans. Rather, it was first developed by single-cellular microbes and was worked on and advanced by many different forms of life predating humans, and eventually we inherited this gift—our innate immune system. It comes pre-programmed to recognize threats and remove them based upon experience and intelligence evolved over billions of years. Stop for a moment and think about that, because this is far beyond any human invention ever created. Nature is much smarter and wiser than we are.

But there's a problem. The microbes are little shape-shifters. They can change and adapt extremely quickly. For example, if you give a person antibiotics, they will evolve antibiotic resistance almost immediately. The way this happens is that most microbes are killed by the antibiotics, but the ones that survive have the resistance gene and no competition for resources. This leads to massive and rapid reproduction that could generate up to fifty new generations in one turn of the sun. In just eleven days they can evolve a thousandfold increase in antibiotic resistance. This is their superpower. Single-celled organisms have evolutionary speed that can leave our innate immune system in the dust.

This is why we evolved our adaptive immune system, which has two much-needed advantages. First, it can change as fast as the microbes do. There's always going to be a delay, because it's reacting. But give it a few days and it will create targeted, precise antibodies. Second, it has a memory that allows it to learn and build upon itself. Over time it becomes faster, stronger, and more decisive.

But importantly, the adaptive immune system does not come pre-programmed in the way that the innate immune system does. At birth, our adaptive immune system is a blank canvas—full of potential, yet untested and untrained for defense. And then moving forward, it learns, it develops progressive knowledge and abilities, and over time it becomes diverse and personalized in much the same way that our gut microbiome is diverse and personalized. And much like the gut microbiome, it is diversity within the adaptive immune system that in fact gives it its strength and power. But in order for the adaptive immune system to mature to its full potential, it must be trained and mentored. A diverse immune system is built by exposure to a diverse mix of microbes—bacteria, yeast, parasites, archaea, and viruses. The broader the exposure, the better the training, because it creates more experience for the adaptive immune system, more opportunity to learn. This allows it to more effectively discriminate friend from foe and develop a bigger arsenal that is ready to protect and defend us. But where might we find such a mix of microbes?

Our adaptive immune system is perhaps the most important part of our bodily defenses. An infant born with a defective adaptive immune system will not survive very long. But we really, really trust our gut microbes, and this is evidenced by the fact that we evolved an adaptive immune system that is educated by those microbes. It is an example of co-evolution. Over millennia, we co-evolved with our microbes to have an adaptive immune system that stands in defense of our body. And during the course of our lifetime, we refine our own personal adaptive immune system with the help of our gut microbes so that it as dynamic, as unique, as diverse, and as powerful as possible.

Nurtured by Nature from Conception Through Life's Stages

Let's consider the many ways microbes nurture the development of a baby during pregnancy and infancy. Mom's gut microbiome changes during pregnancy to facilitate weight gain and make sure both mom and baby have what they need to grow. Meanwhile, those microbes produce chemicals, such as short-chain fatty acids, that cross the placenta and influence immune development in the baby. As the pregnancy progresses, microbes cross the placenta to colonize the baby's gut and start training the immune system. Then, during the third trimester, mom's vaginal microbiome changes to prepare for the baby to pass through the birth canal, receive the gift of microbes, and seed the newborn's gut with the right microbes to support its early life needs. This is why cesarean delivery has been associated with less gut diversity and an increased risk of allergic, autoimmune, and metabolic diseases in the baby.

Next up is mom's breast milk, which contains microbes, short-chain fatty acids, a variety of antibodies to target and eliminate pathogens, and two hundred varieties of human milk oligosaccharides, which are prebiotics to feed and fuel the baby's developing gut microbiome. Breast milk is nature's gut and immune health drink. This is why breastfeeding is associated with a lower risk of allergic, autoimmune, and metabolic diseases in the baby. These are just some examples of how the gut microbes support and nurture from the moment of conception, through pregnancy and our childhood and continuing through all of life's stages all the way to the finish line. These are our life partners, and if we take care of them, they will take care of us.

When Barriers Break and LPS Gets Unleashed on the Body

These historical connections bring us forward to today—right here, right now. What happens when our defenses fail and LPS crosses the gut barrier? That's the real question, especially in light of our immune system's ancient origins. Let's pull out our microscope again and take a closer look.

LPS isn't supposed to be in the blood. That's why we have a gut barrier, to keep the pathogenic bacteria out. But if LPS crosses the gut barrier, your immune system recognizes its age-old enemy and goes to war, which is inflammation. A small amount of LPS leads to a skirmish, or low-grade inflammation. A large amount of LPS leads to sepsis, which is what you see happening in the hospital intensive care unit with people who are on life support.

Inflammation always comes with a price. When it's low-grade inflammation, the number one symptom is fatigue. There's always fatigue. Inflammation is energy zapping. But there might also be brain fog, body aches and joint pains, weight gain, higher blood sugar, rashes, gum disease and bad breath, anxiousness or feeling down, messed-up appetite, poor sleep, or, of course, gut symptoms. These are the day-to-day manifestations of a broken gut barrier that's leaking LPS, resulting in chronic low-grade inflammation, which also leads to all of the health conditions that I shared with you in the beginning of the book.

When it's high-grade inflammation, such as in sepsis, the price is organ failure. The way this happens is that inflammation actually destroys tight junctions. These junctions hold your gut barrier together. They hold your brain barrier together. They also hold your blood vessels together. Your body is compartmentalized to keep each important part of it safe, but when the immune system goes to war, it releases chemicals, such as histamine, that disrupt the tight junctions and break down these barriers. The result is leakage. When there's inflammation in your nose from seasonal allergies, the leakage results in a runny nose. But in sepsis the leakage happens through the entire body, resulting in multiorgan failure—brain, lungs, heart, kidneys, liver. This is how people can go from developing a urinary tract infection, pneumonia, or COVID to multiorgan failure and fighting for their life in the hospital.

LPS is pure gasoline on the flames of inflammation. And while we definitely want to avoid a nuclear meltdown, it's the day-to-day seepage of LPS that quietly saps our energy, clouds our thinking, and sets the stage for more serious issues. The truth is, it's neither possible nor necessary to eliminate every trace of LPS. Our real goal is to strengthen our defenses—shoring up the gut barrier and keeping LPS locked inside the intestines so the immune system can maintain its calm, focused vigilance.

Extinguishing the Flames Within: Rebalancing Your Inner Ecosystem

So, how do we make those defenses stronger? Now that we see how inflammation occurs on a microscopic level, let's zoom out to view its effects on your body as a whole and how understanding this big picture can help you keep it in check.

Imagine that your body is a vast, expansive forest. It's beautiful—teeming with life that all functions in harmonious balance. Sure, the forest accumulates some dead leaves and fallen trees from time to time, but in general, it is a lush, thriving ecosystem, home to a diverse variety of forest creatures, everything from the smallest insect to the tall, ancient trees.

Every now and then, lightning strikes in the forest, setting off a fire. This fire clears out the deadwood and burns out quickly, making way for new growth. It's contained and self-limited, and helps keep the forest healthy. This is like the acute inflammation that your body experiences after an injury or during an infection. This type of inflammation serves a purpose and is short-lived. But if the conditions in the forest are not healthy, if they include deforestation, the introduction of invasive species, pollution, soil erosion, or a major storm, the forest's balance is chronically disrupted. The result is a shift toward more fallen trees and more leaves on the forest floor. There is more fuel for a forest fire.

In our body, a nutrient-poor diet, toxins, a dysfunctional lifestyle, and stress are the conditions that create the fuel for the flames of inflammation. When the fire starts, we have a huge problem. It isn't controlled and self-limited. It is out of control and looking to spread. The fire burns higher and hotter, inflicting collateral harm to life in our forest. This is what happens in septic shock when an infection spins out of control and the problem stops being the virus and starts being the immune system. It's the same problem with allergic and autoimmune diseases, where the immune system is viciously attacking something completely friendly and benign. And this is also what happens with chronic low-grade inflammation, where the continual activation of the immune system leads to progressive scars that manifest with aging and disease. Over time, this smoldering inflammation damages blood vessels, laying the groundwork for atherosclerosis and heart disease. It drives uncontrolled cell signaling and DNA damage, increasing the risk of cancer. It wears down insulin sensitivity, setting the stage for type 2 diabetes. It even disrupts brain function, contributing to neurodegenerative conditions like Alzheimer's disease and Parkinson's disease. Low-grade inflammation is the common thread linking modern chronic diseases, turning the body's defense system into a slow-burning fire that weakens us over time.

In nature, an unchecked forest fire creates new problems—habitat destruction, biodiversity loss, air pollution, and water pollution, to name a few. In our body, chronic inflammation creates its own cascade of harm—organ damage, impaired physiology, and gut microbiome injury. This sets off a chain reaction because the gut microbiome is connected to so many other aspects of our health, including our digestion, immune system, metabolism, hormones, and cognitive health. There's also the consequences of inflammation on how we feel—our energy levels, mood, gut symptoms, hunger, menopause or menstrual comfort, mental clarity, and other physical symptoms.

We have firefighters to fight forest fires—and thank goodness for that. But just because we have them doesn't mean we should accept every blaze as inevitable or allow forests to burn unchecked. We also have doctors, nurses, and other health care workers to help us fight the flames of inflammation. But that doesn't mean we should wait until we have serious health problems and then expect them to clean up the mess. Sometimes, despite their best efforts, the fire still burns higher and hotter.

Why can't they catch up to it and put it out? Because the forest is constantly fueling its own destruction with a buildup of deadwood—just as our bodies can fuel inflammation with nutrient-poor diets, toxins, stress, and other factors. You might slow the flames in one area, but new tinder quickly ignites elsewhere, faster than medical interventions can stamp them out. We're caught in a losing battle when all we do is chase fires as they flare.

So do we give up on conventional medicine? Absolutely not. We'd be far worse off without it. But we need to take responsibility for our own forest. The choices that we make can prevent fires altogether, or at least make them easier to handle. We can support our health care heroes by addressing the bigger picture. That starts with answering two urgent questions:

1. What's the actual source of our problem?

2. What factors exist that we can control to protect ourselves—now and in the future?

Ultimately, the best approach is to prevent the blaze altogether—or at least limit its impact as much as possible—by reducing the nutrient-poor diets, toxins, dysfunctional lifestyles, and stress that make us vulnerable. Each of these factors fuels inflammation. Tackling only one is like dousing a single hot spot, barely making a dent—but addressing them all can massively undermine the entire fire. We want to get the forest back to its lush, expansive, diverse, healthy state. A thriving forest means a thriving ecosystem where the life within it benefits. The way that we accomplish this is by controlling the factors that facilitate health within the ecosystem.

The Environment Shapes the Organism

There's an equilibrium within an ecosystem. Call it balance or harmony. Of course, change is inevitable. It requires adjustment by life within an ecosystem. Small changes require small adaptations. But when there are major disruptions, we lose the ability to adapt.

In Chapter 1, I mentioned the word that best describes this—"dysbiosis." Dysbiosis is a diseased ecosystem that's failing. The environment has changed and the ecosystem no longer fits. To heal, we need to restore the environment that previously allowed it to thrive and bring back the biodiversity that, by design, will get things working again.

We have the ability to control all the factors and create powerful and transformative healing. We just need to see the bigger picture, the forest for the trees. The environment shapes the organism. Ecosystems evolve to fit the environment. Individual organisms evolve to fit their ecosystem.

This is a law of nature that was true billions of years ago, is equally true today, and will be true tomorrow. What's exciting is that YOU have the ability to create the environment when it's your gut. YOU create the conditions. Without awareness about the way this works, you simply float along doing the wildly abnormal things that we have normalized in our society—eating convenient ultra-processed foods that starve your gut microbes, living a sedentary lifestyle that slows gut motility, enjoying the comforts of your home that deprive you of sun and nature, prioritizing stress and hustle over rest and recovery, shining bright lights in our face after the sun goes down, and getting by with crappy sleep while wondering why you feel exhausted and inflamed. These behaviors feel "normal" because they are common, but they are completely out of sync with how we evolved to interact with our environment. But the truth is we can hack the laws of nature to create an environment that heals our gut microbiome, our immune system, and ultimately us.

All life is forced to adapt to its environment in an effort to survive. That's evolution. It's been that way since the beginning and remains that way today. We learned to survive and thrive with our gut microbes. They were a part of our story and remain essential to our health.

Our microbes are evolving as we speak. This is their superpower—rapid evolution. Imagine if in just eleven days you could develop a new attribute that makes you a thousand times stronger, smarter, or more resilient. Yeah, we can't do that. Our microbes can, though.

Humans have a different superpower. Through the powers of human intelligence, we have the ability to alter and manipulate our environment. Even more powerfully, we have the ability to control the environment in which our microbes live, through our food and lifestyle choices. This is a godlike superpower.

But what happens if the alterations and manipulations of our environment are made without the microbes in mind? What if we have different motivations—say, convenience or comfort or some form of satisfaction? Our technology could be our greatest power. It also has the potential to be our downfall if our innovation and lifestyle are disconnected from the needs and historical origins of us and our microbes.

Chapter 2 is backed by 84 references gathered through an extensive review of the scientific literature. You can browse the full citation list at www .theguthealthmd.com/plantpoweredplus.

TOXIC ENVIRONMENTS

The Price We Pay to Be Evolutionary Pioneers

There were consistent patterns to the way we lived as humans for millions of years. We ate real food, walked to get around, rose with the sun and rested with the moon, and invested heavily in interpersonal connection. But the problem we have as a species is that our intelligence facilitates innovation and control over our environment. Our greatest strength is our biggest weakness because it seduces us. We can't resist it. Next thing you know, we are evolutionary pioneers, drifting farther and farther from the trail that was blazed by our ancestors before us.

Over the last two hundred years our diet has undergone a radical transformation as science and technology developed new ways to preserve, prepare, reconfigure, synthetically fertilize, genetically modify, and mass-produce our food. For one thing, instead of growing produce ourselves, foraging, or buying from a local farmer, we now source the overwhelming majority of our fresh food from supermarkets that sell food several steps removed from their origin. Fruits and vegetables are harvested by a machine, cleaned and sorted on a conveyor belt, sprayed with chemicals to enhance their shelf life, packaged in plastic and shipped through a network of warehouses and distribution centers, and eventually arrive at a grocery store, where they sit on the shelves.

But we've taken a step further with food that is so technologically altered that it barely resembles its origins in nature. The idea of milling a grain to produce flour has been around for a long time, but in the twentieth century, the exponential growth of technology was paralleled by the development of food science. I'm not talking about nutritional science, which is the study of how food impacts human health and well-being; I'm talking about food science—a new field intending to create new foods or extend the shelf life of our current foods. The focus is on the creation of food, not on nutrition. As a result, a new wave of foods came on the market—canned and processed meats, sugary breakfast cereals, white bread, sweetened drinks and sauces, and frozen dinners.

There are upsides to all of this innovation—less spoilage and waste, more calories with less cost, less hunger and food insecurity, food with flavors and qualities that we enjoy, and, most important, convenience. These are desirable outcomes, no? But all this evolutionary pioneering is not without a downside. Remember that we spent millions if not billions of years co-evolving with our microbes. We had a long-established relationship with biological processes that worked—our genome adapted to them. Rather than honor those connections, the modern diet and lifestyle upend that relationship by moving in a direction we've never taken before. The result is that we become incompatible with our own biology. This is perhaps nowhere more evident than in our gut.

Our modern choices have led us down a road of convenient, lab-altered, mass-produced foods and a chronically stressful lifestyle. The result is a toxic disconnect between our biology and our environment, one that weakens our gut microbes, erodes our gut barrier, and overloads our immune system with perpetual low-level inflammation. Thankfully, we're too resilient for this to end us on the spot—but it's enough to drain our energy, dull our vitality, and slowly suck away our health. So, what exactly are these modern foods, farming practices, and lifestyle factors doing to our bodies—and is there a way back to harmony with our biology? Let's take a closer look.

Down on the Farm

Gone is the idyllic farm of our grandparents or great-grandparents. They were sanctuaries for nature and the rhythm of the seasons, with sprawling rows of varied crops swaying under the nourishing sun. And they were a multigenerational legacy for a family that works hard and appreciates the land and what it provides. Today's industrialized modern farm is a mechanized operation, prioritizing efficiency and maximum yields, preferring monoculture fields and large-scale animal feeding operations, all managed with the aid of technological intrusions, advanced chemicals, and synthetic inputs.

New innovations emerge. Consolidation occurs around the new technology. Scale and efficiency improve. The short-term gains are readily apparent in the financial books. The CEO gets a juicy bonus and the shareholders are happy. But as smart as this formula seems, it's missing something really, really important but not immediately obvious. In our haste to pursue rapid gains, we've lost sight of the fact that farming is a delicate dance among soil, microbes, and the broader ecosystem in which they exist. We are disrupting the balance of nature and causing mass-scale dysbiosis. When the microbial world is thrown off-kilter, the consequences inevitably ripple up the food chain, ultimately affecting our own health.

This is most exemplified in the tragic tale of greed and gluttony in the use of glyphosate, just one example of how our modern farming practices are disconnected from our health. Glyphosate was discovered in 1970 as a broad-spectrum herbicide. That means it kills plants. And I'm pretty sure you get what broad spectrum means.

Glyphosate started as a weed killer. You've surely seen it and possibly used it in your yard as Roundup, which is glyphosate combined with various adjuvants to make it an even stronger weed killer. At first you could spray it only where you wanted to kill all the vegetation. In the 1990s it became popular as a desiccant, which means that when you harvest a crop and need to dry it out, you can accelerate that process by spraying it with glyphosate. This is most applicable to cereal grains (wheat and oats) as well as dried legumes (beans, lentils, and peas). If you spray a field with glyphosate, some of the plants will have genes that make them glyphosate resistant, much like the way antibiotic-resistant microbes thrive when we use antibiotics. In 1995, Monsanto figured out how to genetically engineer plants that were preferentially glyphosate tolerant. Over the coming years, "Roundup Ready" GMO soy, corn, cotton, alfalfa, and sugar beets were developed. More recently, Roundup Ready grass helped create the beautiful yards that children and dogs play in. If you're keeping tabs, glyphosate is now widely used for agriculture (that we eat) as well as commercial, industrial, and residential areas. I should mention that glyphosate is extremely cheap, averaging between one dollar and thirteen dollars per acre of spray. This is how glyphosate became the most used herbicide in the world—280 million pounds sprayed per year in the United States alone. Because glyphosate is water-soluble, it lingers in waterways, which is why it's now often detected in our water, soil, food, and even human urine.

Glyphosate blocks an enzyme in what's called the shikimate pathway, which is how plants and microorganisms create amino acids like tryptophan, tyrosine, and phenylalanine. Tryptophan is the precursor to serotonin, the happy hormone. More on that in Chapter 6. Animals are not reliant on the shikimate pathway, so Monsanto argued that there are no consequences for humans from exposure to glyphosate. But if glyphosate kills plants by blocking the shikimate pathway, what do we suppose happens to microbes that are also reliant on the shikimate pathway? By targeting this pathway, glyphosate inadvertently disrupts microbial communities that are crucial not only to soil fertility but also to our gut health.

Some of them, like *Staph aureus* and *Strep pneumoniae* (the causes of skin and lung infections), are naturally more glyphosate tolerant. Others, like *E. coli*, can develop mutations to protect themselves. Advantageous mutations seem to preferentially occur with the pathogenic microbes, meaning they are more likely to survive glyphosate exposure. The very organisms that we most want to keep in check may be the first to adapt and thrive when exposed to glyphosate. Meanwhile, even low-dose glyphosate exposure depletes the body of beneficial microbes like *Bifidobacterium* and *Lactobacillus*. In animal models, long-term exposure to very small amounts of Roundup altered tight junction proteins and damaged the gut barrier. This activates the immune system to cause inflammation.

Of course, there are consequences to this. And we're just beginning to learn exactly what they are. Glyphosate is an endocrine disrupter, which means that it throws normal hormonal balance out of whack through inhibition of estrogen production in the placenta and baby embryo, simultaneous activation of estrogen receptors, and reduced testosterone production. Even at low doses this may affect female fertility. Exposure to Roundup is associated with anxiety and depression in mice. It's been associated with ADHD and autism-spectrum disorders (ASDs) in humans. There are concerns that it is altering thyroid function. Some believe glyphosate is responsible for the rise of celiac disease. The science is evolving, but the emerging themes raise concerns about glyphosate's far-reaching impacts on both our bodies and the broader environment. Yet none of this appears on food labels—"sprayed with glyphosate" is nowhere to be found. At the very least, we deserve transparency so that anyone who wants to avoid it has the information to do so.

The issues that exist with our modern farming practices are exemplified by but not limited to glyphosate. A good first step in the pursuit of healthier food would be to nurture healthier soil, where most of our nutrients originate. When we acknowledge and care for our soil, we are restoring healthy microbes in the soil, the plants that it produces, and the humans who are fed. Regenerative farming techniques can help restore this delicate balance. This is not just a problem for our farmers. It is our responsibility to reconnect with the land and honor the connections among soil, microbes, and our well-being.

Modern Farming Practices and Animal Products

Speaking of the issues that exist in our modern farming practices, consider what we've done to animals. Yes, there are ethical issues that exist around how the animals are treated, but let's put that to the side for a moment. Much as the human diet and lifestyle have radically changed in the last hundred years, so too has life radically changed for livestock. Take the cow, for example. Once free-range and grass-fed, it now spends most—or all—of its life stressed out in concentrated animal feeding operations (CAFOs), packed tightly with thousands of other cattle with no room to move. Instead of grazing on nutrient-rich pastures, it's fed a grain-based diet, primarily consisting of genetically modified corn and soy. That corn and soy have often been sprayed with glyphosate, such that glyphosate residues are detectable in cows' meat and milk. Beyond diet, modern cows are routinely given antibiotics to prevent disease in their over-crowded conditions, as well as growth hormones to maximize production. The cow has been totally removed from its natural diet, natural habitat, and natural lifestyle. And we do similar things to pigs and chickens. We've come a long way from the days where the animal products in our diet were wild animals that lived healthy lives within a balanced ecosystem. If our food is sick, how can it make us healthy?

The Big Three: Sugar, Fat, and Salt

We are evolutionarily motivated to seek sweet, salty, and fatty foods. Sugar is energy for physical and mental activity. Your brain requires glucose (sugar) as its fuel. Fats make up most of the mass of the brain and provide more than twice as many calories, gram for gram, when compared to proteins and carbohydrates. Sugar and fat were efficient sources of energy in times of food scarcity and famine. We seek salt because sodium is an essential nutrient that was in short supply in most environments. Evolving in times of food scarcity, we developed a deeply embedded preference for sugar, fat, and salt that guided us toward survival in the past, but now that we can consume them to total excess, they are destroying our gut, creating inflammation, and shortening our life expectancy.

We avoid bitter flavors because sometimes that indicates poison. In ancient times, we didn't have *The Farmer's Almanac* to guide our food choices, just our senses and gut instincts. If you chose poorly, you either learned fast or didn't survive to choose again. Survival of the fittest was brutal. The irony is that many bitter compounds in plants—like polyphenols—are profoundly beneficial, even though we've evolved to treat bitterness with suspicion.

Our preference for sugar, fat, and salt is more than a mere liking. It even goes beyond genetic programming or a compulsion. There's a reason why eating these nutrients gives you a short-lived rush of feeling fantastic, followed by a crash that leaves you craving another bump. If it sounds like what illicit drugs do, it should, because it's quite similar. Much like addictive drugs, these so-called hyper-palatable foods are associated with obsession, relapse, unintended overconsumption, and impaired control.

What many don't realize is that hyper-palatable foods aren't an accident. Food scientists have figured out that combining two of the Big Three—sugar and fat, salt and carbs, or fat and salt—creates a flavor bomb that lights up your brain's reward centers. That hook keeps you coming back, shuffling into the supermarket for your food fix. Some argue that "food addiction" doesn't exist, but I'm not sure why. It seems obvious when so many of us have trouble ditching these foods. I sure did, fifteen years ago, when I was fifty pounds overweight, depressed, anxious, and metabolically off track, and my gut was a mess. I'm grateful those days are behind me, but if I'd only stuck with what medical school taught me—never connecting my diet, my gut microbes, and my overall health—I'd probably still be riding the junk-food roller coaster.

But the trouble doesn't stop at extra flavor—combining two of the Big Three also amplifies the harm. For instance, if you feed a mouse a high-fat, high-sugar diet, their microbiome suffers, their gut barrier weakens, and inflammation goes into overdrive. They rise and fall together:

BROKEN BIOME + BROKEN BARRIER = INFLAMMATION

But there are further consequences, because this damage alters neurotransmitter levels in the gut, which then impacts the brain, changing the way the brain works. Scientists often discuss the gut-brain axis, referring to how changes in gut health can directly impact brain function and mental health, and vice versa. We'll be digging into this in great detail in Chapter 8 to explore how we can manipulate the brain-gut-immune triangle to our advantage, but what we are seeing here is our first example of these connections.

Research in humans shows that high intake of added sugar and unhealthy fat alters brain function, impairs memory, fosters impulsive food choices, and even makes it hard to tell the difference between hunger and satiety. Ever felt compelled to eat junk food and wondered why you were even eating it, unsure of whether you're hungry, bored, or just eating for the sake of eating? This is your brain on junk food. Let's take a closer look at these three modern culprits.

Sugar and Your Microbiome

It's scary what just a couple of days of sugar does to the microbiome. A recent study started with healthy people who were eating a high-fiber diet and had no gut symptoms and a generally healthy gut microbiome.

My people! But then they dropped their fiber intake and increased their sugar intake. In just seven days—*seven measly days*—these people experienced a loss of gut diversity and an increase in gut permeability. They developed new symptoms—mostly bloating and abdominal pain. But when they resumed their high-fiber diet, their digestive issues went away.

It's not just the amount of sugar that you eat that matters. What also matters is how high your sugar levels get in your blood. This is something that people with diabetes measure throughout the day to fine-tune their insulin use. More recently, we've had the ability to use devices like a continuous glucose monitor to measure our blood sugar levels in real time. This is potentially valuable because high blood sugar damages the tight junctions and disrupts the gut barrier, promoting leaky gut. This may help explain why people with type 2 diabetes are at greater risk for Alzheimer's disease, female infertility, low testosterone in men, major depression, and severe COVID-19. Or that people with diabetes and inflammatory bowel disease (IBD) are hospitalized more and have more infections than those who have IBD without diabetes.

Health Conditions Associated with Increased Sugar Intake

Crohn's disease	Psoriasis	Menopausal symptoms	Obesity
Ulcerative colitis	Lupus	High blood pressure	Heart attack
Rheumatoid arthritis	Small intestinal bacterial overgrowth (SIBO)	High cholesterol	Stroke
Multiple sclerosis		Diabetes	

What About Carbs?

If you're reading this and immediately want to shout, "Those damn carbs!" I totally get it. Damn those carbs! But at the same time, not all carbs are created equal. There are good carbs and bad carbs. The good ones are complex carbohydrates that include things like fiber and resistant starches that you'll find in beans or whole grains. They're slow to digest, or, in many cases, they end up as food for our microbiome, which we call prebiotic. They stand in contrast to refined carbohydrates, which basically refer to added sugars and flour. Those are our bad carbs. They're fast to digest, spiking our blood sugar at first and then plummeting it a few hours later as we suffer with fatigue. My goal is to get you healthier, and what matters is the quality of the carbs. We can improve the quality of the carbs in your diet by shifting as many refined carbs over to complex carbs as possible.

Unhealthy Fats and Immune System Activation

There are good fats and bad fats, and I definitely am not here to say that all fats are bad. There are many versions of healthy diets, and they all include fat on some level because it is a required dietary nutrient. You would be horribly unhealthy without fat in your diet. What matters is the quality of the fats. You want more of the good ones, less of the bad ones. We'll discuss the good ones in Chapter 5, but let's start with the baddies.

Trans fats. Everyone agrees that trans fats are unhealthy. Literally everyone. They are the worst of the worst. There's no healthy amount of trans fats. In short, they're a dysbiosis and inflammation bomb that is so powerfully connected to heart disease and other health issues that our regulatory bodies did something very rare and took them off the market. In 2021 the Food and Drug Administration revoked the approval for partially hydrogenated oils, the main dietary source of trans fats, which were found in vegetable shortening and stick margarine as well as many ultra-processed foods. Unfortunately, the FDA left a loophole in place. Fully hydrogenated oils are still allowed to be used in manufacturing, such that up to half a gram of trans fats per serving could be included, and, much like glyphosate, they're not even required to report it on the packaging. How about that! At a minimum it's deceptive, and I'm not sure how the FDA could ever justify allowing such deception when their job is to protect us, although I suspect they're not used to being called out in books. I should mention that you'll also find trans fats in some animal products. For example, a cup of whole cow's milk has about 0.2 grams of trans fat. Both industrially produced and naturally sourced trans fats are equally unhealthy, and whenever possible we should avoid them.

Saturated fats. The average American consumes 10,439 grams of saturated fat per year. For my math nerds, that's 10.4 kilos, or 23 pounds, of not just fat but pure saturated fat. This is mainly driven by our consumption of meat and dairy products. According to the USDA, the average American consumes the equivalent of 653 pounds of milk products per year, including 41.7 pounds of cheese and 18.9 pounds of ice cream. That's just dairy. The average American consumes 223 pounds of meat per year, including beef, pork, and poultry. To put this into perspective, the average American man and woman weighs 200 and 171 pounds, respectively. We're eating more than our body weight in meat and triple our body weight in milk products.

But animal products aren't the only source of saturated fats. Coconut and palm oil are a major source of plant-based saturated fat, and they're everywhere. Many food companies even advertise their product as containing coconut oil, which is quite audacious considering what we know about saturated fats.

There's an interesting connection between saturated fat and lipopolysaccharide, the bacterial armor worn by pathogens that triggers inflammation if the pathogens get beyond the gut barrier. As we've discussed, your immune cells are preprogrammed to recognize LPS.

When this happens, your immune system gets activated and inflammation ensues. "Lipo" means fat. Lipopolysaccharide is built on a backbone of saturated fat, and it turns out that it's the saturated fat that the immune system recognizes and reacts to. In fact, if your immune system comes across excessive amounts of saturated fat, it will react the same way—activate, release cytokines, and create inflammation.

As we know from Chapter 2, inflammation damages tight junctions and breaks down barriers. When you consume excess saturated fat, it's the gut barrier that suffers. There are consequences after just one meal, and over time, the impact gets worse. Short term: A single serving of cream—mostly saturated fat—spikes blood lipopolysaccharide levels by 40 percent within just five hours. Medium term: Just five days of a high-saturated-fat, animal-based diet increases the growth of *Bilophila wadsworthia* and *Alistipes putredinis*—microbes linked to increased risk of inflammatory bowel disease and colorectal cancer. Long term: Excessive saturated fat intake triggers chronic inflammatory pathways and explains the link between excessive red meat intake and risks of ulcerative colitis, rheumatoid arthritis, and multiple sclerosis. People seem to have big feelings about saturated fat. It's a nutrition lightning rod. But this really isn't about feelings. It's about the weight of the evidence, which says that excessive saturated fat is bad for our gut.

This isn't to say that you are unhealthy if you have saturated fat in your diet. We all have saturated fat in our diet, and there's no such thing as a zero saturated fat diet. My argument isn't for zero saturated fat. I'm arguing for a better balance and that we dial back the things that we overconsume and dial up the things that are missing. In this case, we need to both reduce our saturated fat intake and increase our fiber intake. But increasing fiber is the crucial piece. In one study, a breakfast that included egg and sausage muffin sandwiches and two hash browns increased LPS levels by 58 percent and TNF-α by 114 percent. No surprises there. The interesting part was that by simply adding fiber, the LPS and TNF-α rise was effectively blocked. Even if we don't reduce our saturated fat intake, we can do a lot of good if we optimize our fiber intake.

Fat and Antibiotic Resistance

Interestingly, in the five-day study I mentioned on the opposite page, in which participants were given meals high in animal-based saturated fat, researchers also found that antibiotic resistance was apparent in the gut. Why would this be? It's not that animal-based foods inherently create antibiotic resistance, but if you treat the animal with antibiotics it will store residues of those antibiotics in its meat, meaning muscle. This is disturbing when you consider that about 80 percent of antibiotics sold in the United States are for use in animal agriculture and not for humans.

Heating fats to high temperatures. In addition to trans and saturated fats, the way you cook any fat can be a problem for your gut health. Heating oil to high temperatures, as is done with frying, leads to oxidation of the fats and cholesterol to create toxic by-products. This is particularly problematic among vegetable oils that are mostly unsaturated fat, but it occurs with all oils upon heating. In a study of 862 French people, fried food was associated with lower gut diversity. By the way, so were sugary drinks, processed meats, and fatty sweets. In a different study among 2,289 people with Crohn's disease, fried chicken was associated with lower gut diversity and reduced levels of fourteen anti-inflammatory, beneficial microbes. Fried food tastes great and is inexpensive, and then you pay the price on the back end with your health.

What About Seed Oils and Omega-6 PUFAs?

In recent years, many have targeted seed oils—like canola, sunflower, grapeseed, safflower, soybean, and corn oils—as the primary villain in our modern health crisis. Seed oils are high in polyunsaturated fatty acids, or PUFAs. There are two main types of PUFAs—omega-3s and omega-6s. Omega-6s have developed a reputation for being inflammatory based upon mechanistic studies. But are they really? This label primarily stems from laboratory research that doesn't always reflect the complexity of real diets.

To understand the bigger picture, let's look at what the science actually shows. In mice, soybean oil (a seed oil high in PUFAs) and olive oil (high in monounsaturated fats, or MUFAs) increased gut diversity, increased beneficial bacteria levels, and improved insulin sensitivity. By contrast, coconut oil—mostly saturated fat—reduced gut diversity, increased LPS levels ninefold, promoted fatty liver, and increased fat production. Among people with Crohn's disease, vegetable oil use actually lowered measures of gut inflammation. Human clinical trials show that saturated fats increase LPS levels in the blood, while PUFAs (including omega-6s) were protective and lowered LPS. Of course, LPS translates into inflammation. In multiple studies, when PUFAs are used instead of saturated fat, inflammation levels actually go down. If it's a question of which fat is more inflammatory, the science says it's saturated fat.

Hear me out, though, because seed oils aren't off the hook, nor am I advocating for the inclusion of seed oils in your diet. We need clarity on why they can be problematic. First, overeating seed oils can lead to weight gain and higher body fat—both inherently inflammatory conditions—because these oils are hyper calorie-dense and have zero fiber. Second, when delicate polyunsaturated fats are heated to extreme temperatures, they produce harmful oxidation by-products, which contribute to oxidative stress in the body. If you must cook at high heat, refined avocado oil offers more stable monounsaturated fats and a higher smoke point. Third, seed oils are often found in ultra-processed foods that also contain a multitude of additives, refined sugars, and flavor enhancers—all of which can harm our gut microbiome. Removing seed oils alone won't magically transform junk food into health food.

Since this is such a hot and controversial topic, let me summarize my thoughts on seed oils. We're overconsuming omega-6 PUFAs, so we should be looking to reduce them and bring them into balance. There are much better options—extra-virgin olive oil at room temperature and refined avocado oil (not extra-virgin) when you cook at a high heat, though we should limit fried foods. Research comparing saturated fats and omega-6 PUFAs generally indicates that saturated fat is more inflammatory, challenging the notion that all seed oils are automatically worse. Yes, we should stop frying with seed oils. But no, we should not replace them with beef tallow. That's rearranging chairs on the *Titanic*. Let's not pretend there's a way to make deep-fried foods healthy; there's not. The reality is that we're overdoing *both* saturated fat and omega-6 PUFAs. A better approach is to replace *both of them* with healthier fats (like omega-3s and monounsaturated fats) and, even better, add more fiber. Let's get back to balance!

Salt: The Good Bacteria Killer

Ninety percent of Americans consume more salt than recommended. This is the result of ultra-processed and restaurant foods that exploit our love for salt to bring us back for more. These foods may contain literally one hundred times more salt when compared to similar home-made meals. I honestly don't understand the obsession with salt-based electrolyte drinks. Sure, they taste good, but the average person already consumes about 3,600 milligrams of sodium per day—well above the recommended *limit* of 2,300 milligrams. Adding just one electrolyte drink, which can contain around 1,000 milligrams of sodium, pushes daily intake to 4,600 milligrams—double the recommended amount. Is that balance? Nope! If our goal is to moderate the things that we are overconsuming, we need to rethink our electrolyte drink obsession.

There are consequences to our choices. It comes as no surprise that excess salt kills bacteria. By creating a highly osmotic environment, salt draws water out of cells—beneficial or otherwise—causing them to shrivel and die. That's why it's used to preserve food. In the gut, this excess salt depletes beneficial *Lactobacillus* species by up to 90 percent, disrupts short-chain fatty acid levels, and triggers immune cells (Th17) linked to autoimmune disease. This explains the associations between salt intake and rheumatoid arthritis, multiple sclerosis, lupus, Crohn's disease, and ulcerative colitis.

There is a normal amount of salt intake that is ideal, and when we're in that window, salt is in no way the problem. In fact, inadequate salt intake can be dangerous, resulting in electrolyte imbalances with potential for heart abnormalities, brain swelling, seizures, coma, and death. But inadequate salt intake outside of having a serious medical issue is very rare. Again, it's important to find balance and ideally hit a salt intake level of 1,500–2,300 milligrams of sodium per day. People who sweat a lot, whether it be through exercise or while at work, will need more. That's when electrolyte beverages may make sense, but let's not get carried away with it.

Should I Eliminate Fermented Foods Due to Their Salt Content?

The answer is no. We will get into fermented foods more in Chapter 5, but the key here is the nuance of salt. Salt is not inherently bad. It's a matter of finding balance and avoiding excess. Fermented foods are not the reason for our excessive salt intake; ultra-processed foods are. And as we will discuss, there are amazing qualities to fermented foods that make it so that we want to get more of them in our diet. Let's not throw the baby out with the bathwater and restrict anti-inflammatory foods on the basis of salt. Instead, let's eliminate the unnecessary ultra-processed foods, normalize our salt intake, and enjoy fermented foods within the context of balanced salt intake.

The Wild Western Diet

So far, we've been looking at the individual effects of excessive sugar (refined carbs), unhealthy fat, and salt on their own. But what happens if you combine the Big Three to create the ultimate nutritional supervillain? We call that the Western diet.

Research shows the typical Western diet powerfully and negatively damages the gut microbiome, lowers gut diversity, promotes the growth of inflammatory bacteria, increases intestinal permeability, and leads to the release of bacterial endotoxin into the bloodstream, chronically activating the immune system to trigger inflammation. It should come as little surprise that a Western diet has been associated with a myriad of chronic inflammatory conditions. It's easiest for me to just pop them into a table for you. As you will notice, the list of health conditions associated with a Western diet overlaps heavily with the list of health conditions that have been associated with dysbiosis and inflammation found on page 371.

Health Conditions Associated with a Western Diet

AUTOIMMUNE, ALLERGIC, AND HORMONAL CONDITIONS	CARDIOVASCULAR, PULMONARY, AND METABOLIC DISEASES	HORMONAL, COGNITIVE, AND NEUROPSYCHIATRIC CONDITIONS	CANCERS
Crohn's disease	Metabolic syndrome	Migraine headaches	Colorectal cancer
Ulcerative colitis	Obesity	Poor cognitive function	Breast cancer
Rheumatoid arthritis	Type 2 diabetes	Memory impairment	Prostate cancer
Psoriasis	Atherosclerosis	Alzheimer's disease	Lung cancer
Multiple sclerosis	Cardiovascular disease	Insomnia	Chronic lymphocytic leukemia
Celiac disease	Coronary artery disease	Anxiety	
Asthma		Depression	Non-Hodgkin lymphoma
Food allergy	Stroke	Bipolar disorder	Hodgkin lymphoma
Endometriosis	Vascular dysfunction	Parkinson's disease	Multiple myeloma
Polycystic ovary syndrome (PCOS)	Hypertension	ADHD	Liver cancer
	Hyperlipidemia		Endometrial cancer
Premenstrual syndrome	Chronic kidney disease		Ovarian cancer
	Nonalcoholic fatty liver disease		Esophageal squamous cancer
Female infertility			
Male infertility	Cirrhosis		Esophageal adenocarcinoma
Erectile dysfunction	Gout		Melanoma
Low testosterone (hypogonadism)			Stomach cancer
			Thyroid cancer

The Main Culprit of the Western Diet—Ultra-Processed Foods

Picture the scene: Lightning strikes over the food science lab. *"It's alive! It's alive!"* The newest Frankenstein-like food lumbers forward to take its place on our supermarket shelf: "ultra-processed foods," or UPFs. Through intensive processing, the food industry discovered that they could manipulate the sugar, fat, and salt to make foods that create pleasure and hedonia. Researcher and psychophysicist Howard Moskowitz coined the term "bliss point" to describe how UPFs work. What it boils down to is that food manufacturers deliberately create foods that hit our bliss point so that we keep coming back for more.

Ultra-processed foods now make up 73 percent of the US food supply and 57 percent of the calories consumed. Our children get 67 percent of their calories from UPFs. The UK and Canada are not far behind, with 56 percent and 45 percent of consumed calories, respectively, coming from UPFs.

People still need to eat, and let's be honest—UPFs taste good, they're cheap, and they fit our hectic schedules. They align perfectly in our modern world that is fast paced and financially tense. Big Food knows what we want. But they weren't formulated to make you healthier or to support your gut microbiome. Those factors aren't a consideration in this equation.

UPFs aren't just inexpensive, convenient, and tasty. They are also hyper-palatable, meaning they're designed for overconsumption. It's been proven. Dr. Kevin Hall did a fascinating study where he had people living in a research dormitory at the NIH eating two weeks each of a minimally processed versus an ultra-processed diet. The meals were matched for calories, energy density, macronutrients, sugar, sodium, and fiber. No differences there! The participants were told to eat until they were full, so that's what they did. What happened? Participants on the ultra-processed diet ate 508 more kilocalories *per day*. That equates to about a pound of weight gain per week. Over time, these extra calories accumulate, driving weight gain, metabolic issues, and inflammation. Look around you—our stores and pantries are filled with UPFs, and our communities are filled with obesity and chronic disease.

The true price we pay for these foods is not in dollars and cents; it's in years and health. When new products flood our plates, we bear the brunt of their potential harms from the start, often without any

immediate warning signs. It can take years and countless affected individuals before suspicions arise and retrospective epidemiological studies even begin. Even then, pinpointing the exact cause of disease is
incredibly challenging amid thousands of dietary variables consumed
in ever-changing amounts. It's an undeniable mess.

The result is that science is perpetually trying to catch up. We don't
have it all figured out, but we've come a long way. When I wrote *Fiber
Fueled* back in 2019, I shared two references to indicate the health concerns of ultra-processed foods. By the time I wrote *The Fiber Fueled
Cookbook* just two years later, I had twenty-two studies to share. The
health conditions these studies covered included obesity, heart disease,
cancer, stroke, Alzheimer's disease, diabetes, and chronic kidney disease. That's six of the top ten causes of death in the United States.
Here's an important fact that I want you to process for a minute before
you move on: In a prospective cohort study, researchers found that every 10 percent increase in consumption of ultra-processed foods was
associated with a 14 percent risk of early death. Our kids are consuming an almost 70 percent UPF diet, which is some scary math. Basically, if you want to live longer, reduce your intake of UPFs as much as
possible.

As I prepared this book, a massive umbrella review of UPF meta-
analyses was published, covering forty-five adverse health outcomes
among nearly ten million people, including multiple mental health,
cardiovascular, gastrointestinal, metabolic, and respiratory health outcomes as well as seven forms of cancer. The results: Ultra-processed
foods were linked to increased risk of thirty-two different health conditions. Further, forty-two of the forty-five health outcomes showed at
least a trend toward the UPFs being harmful, even if ten of them didn't
meet statistical significance. There's a pattern emerging. Give it time
and let's see where that goes when we have more data.

But what about chronic inflammatory diseases? Ultra-processed food intake has been associated with increased risk of Crohn's disease, ulcerative colitis, multiple sclerosis, lupus, polycystic ovary syndrome, gout, asthma, eczema, and food allergies. In addition, UPFs have been connected to irritable bowel syndrome (IBS), thyroid dysfunction, depression, anxiety, ADHD, and menopausal symptoms. Men who eat more ultra-processed foods have lower sperm counts and lower sperm concentration. In addition, the sperm are slower and more likely to be deformed. I'm speaking for all men when I say: Leave my damn sperm alone!

Let me be clear about where I stand. I'm not arguing that every single UPF is toxic. We don't know that's true and it's not something I believe. What is true is that the dose matters. Even if a food is a problem, having it once is not going to substantially harm you. But over time, you'll experience a real impact. We can't pretend that UPFs are safe for regular consumption like our food industry suggests.

Just like the tobacco industry did in the 1950s and early 1960s, the food industry is actively working to obscure the risks. Big Tobacco created the playbook. They fund research designed to produce favorable results, lobby to have industry-funded studies prioritized over independent research, and create financial ties and dependencies for key stakeholders and trusted thought leaders. They consistently ignore and undermine studies that suggest harm and fund manipulative review articles that dishonestly cherry-pick whatever fits their preferred narrative. They bully and publicly discredit scientists who raise concerns. They lobby and aggressively push back against policies that could regulate harmful additives or excessive processing, making it hard to institute change, and then they purchase influence in mainstream and social media to dominate the propaganda war. They mislead the public with marketing that preys upon our struggles and vulnerabilities, and when challenged, they create doubt, dismiss opposing research, and label critics as alarmists. First it was Big Tobacco; now it's Big Food. History is repeating itself right before our eyes.

The Newest Threat: Microplastics and Nanoplastics—Here's What You Need to Know

Perhaps you've heard of microplastics, which are tiny plastic particles less than 5 millimeters in size. They're piling up in our environment due to pollution and skyrocketing plastic use worldwide, and because many plastics do not fully biodegrade, weathering simply splits them into fragments. While microplastics are concerning, I'm even more alarmed by nanoplastics, which are invisible to the naked eye. Their diminutive size may cause big problems because they can get absorbed, enter cells, and bioaccumulate.

Microplastics and nanoplastics have become pervasive in our environment, infiltrating the air we breathe, the water we drink, and the food we consume. Recent studies have detected nanoplastics in various human tissues, including the brain, liver, kidneys, and lungs, raising concerns about potential health impacts. In one observational study, researchers found plastic particles lodged in plaque within the carotid artery, a major blood vessel in the neck that supplies blood to the brain. Participants with these plastic-containing plaques were more likely to suffer strokes, heart attacks, or death. While definitive human data are just starting to emerge, animal studies suggest possible risks such as inflammation, oxidative stress, disruptions to the reproductive system, and connections to colon cancer and lung cancer. Suffice it to say that there's no possibility that microplastics and nanoplastics are good for us.

That doesn't mean that all plastics are inherently harmful, but certain conditions—like heat or acidity—can increase the risk of toxic chemicals leaching into your food and beverages. To mitigate risk, it's best to avoid anything where heat or acid contact plastic prior to your consumption. Avoid microwaving plastic containers, be cautious with take-out packaging, and don't drink warm beverages or soups from plastic. Coffee drinkers, pause and consider where plastic may exist in your brewer, single-serve pods, or even your cup. Tea drinkers, you're not off the hook—some tea bags contain plastic, too. That also means avoiding tomatoes, sauerkraut, kombucha, or other acidic foods that are more safely stored in glass or stainless steel. Be wary of water or soft drinks in plastic bottles. And speaking of water, consider investing in a reverse osmosis water filtration system that purifies your water, reduces plastic waste and exposure, *and* saves you money in the long run. For more tips on minimizing toxic exposures at home, check page 376 in the Appendix.

Food Additives: The Genie Is Out of the Bottle

The food industry is not the Wild West. We do have rules and government regulation. It's just the lightest, most food-industry-friendly oversight possible. While drug companies must pass through four phases of drug development and spend millions on large human trials, food additives get quick and painless approval through a loophole called "Generally Recognized as Safe," or GRAS.

The GRAS loophole began in 1958 with an amendment to the Federal Food, Drug, and Cosmetic Act to make it easier for common ingredients like flour, salt, and vinegar to get approved as long as a group of experts felt they were safe. Perhaps the impact of this amendment in the future wasn't clear in 1958, nor was it the intent of the law, but it ended up creating the opportunity for exploitation because the food industry could introduce any and all ingredients as GRAS with essentially no oversight. Here's what that looks like:

- **Limited or no feeding studies:** Nearly 80 percent of approved chemicals lack human or even animal model feeding studies to demonstrate safety. Think about that!

- **Short-term data predominates:** When human safety data do exist, they are generally short term. So what happens long term? I guess we're finding out as we go.

- **No microbiome testing requirement:** Although modern science can assess how additives affect our gut microbes, the FDA does not mandate microbiome testing for additives. Yes, microbiome testing is a new technology. But we don't want our regulatory bodies stuck in the 1970s, do we?

- **Lack of systematic reevaluation:** Once an additive is deemed GRAS, there's no formal mechanism that regularly revisits old decisions in light of fresh evidence. An additive approved fifty years ago may never be reevaluated, even if new data emerges.

- **Few or no follow-up studies:** Once an additive is approved, there's no requirement for the food industry to conduct further safety research or monitoring, meaning any long-term risks may go undetected.

- **Scarce independent funding:** Academic researchers generally rely on grants to support their work. With minimal public, industry, or government investment in food additive safety, relatively few experts can explore potential harms. This funding gap perpetuates our knowledge deficit.

So if there's no money in food safety research, but there is tons of money working for Big Food, where do you think the jobs exist, where do the experts make their money, and where do you think loyalty exists? As I often tell my kids, you don't want to bite the hand that feeds you.

On a systemic level, GRAS approval is like a river running down the mountain. There are powerful currents carrying momentum in one direction, and it's really hard to go against that. As a result, you end up with ten thousand approved additives against just thirty-five banned substances. In fact, the rate of substance banning has slowed down dramatically, with just eight substances banned since 1982. It is the system that is creating this imbalance.

Ten thousand additives get dumped into our food supply, consumed by hundreds of millions in varied amounts and intervals over years, and we're expected to figure out which ones specifically are problematic without having the funding to support that level of research. The status quo is pretty easy to maintain when it's nearly impossible to prove harm. They're not *all* dangerous or toxic, but some of them are, and we aren't adequately testing them, monitoring them, or scrutinizing them to know that they are safe for long-term human consumption. Here are a few examples to consider.

Animal Model Effects of Food Additives on Microbiome, Gut Barrier, and Immune System with Human Disease Associations

ADDITIVE TYPE	ADDITIVE EXAMPLES	MICROBIOME EFFECTS	GUT BARRIER EFFECTS	IMMUNE EFFECTS	HUMAN DISEASE CONCERNS
Artificial sweeteners	Aspartame	↓ Diversity ↑ Invasive *E. coli, E. faecalis*	↓ Tight junctions ↑ Permeability	↑ Inflammation ↑ Intestinal inflammation	Cancer Crohn's disease Diabetes Obesity Stroke IBS
	Sucralose	↓ Diversity ↑ *Shigella, Bilophila* ↑ Invasive *E. coli, E. faecalis*	↓ Tight junctions ↑ Permeability	↑ Inflammatory cytokines ↑ Intestinal inflammation	Coronary heart disease Crohn's disease Diabetes IBS
	Saccharin	↑ Dysbiosis ↑ *E. coli* biofilm formation ↑ Invasive *E. faecalis*	↑ Permeability	↑ Inflammation ↑ Intestinal inflammation	Diabetes Liver inflammation
	Acesulfame potassium	↓ Diversity ↑ Dysbiosis	↑ Permeability ↑ Bacterial translocation	↑ Inflammatory cytokines ↑ Intestinal inflammation	Coronary heart disease Diabetes IBS
Emulsifiers	Carboxymethylcellulose (CMC)	↓ Diversity	↓ Mucus layer thickness ↑ Permeability	↑ Intestinal inflammation	Crohn's disease Ulcerative colitis Cardiovascular disease Coronary artery disease Colorectal cancer Obesity IBS

ADDITIVE TYPE	ADDITIVE EXAMPLES	MICROBIOME EFFECTS	GUT BARRIER EFFECTS	IMMUNE EFFECTS	HUMAN DISEASE CONCERNS
Emulsifiers	Polysorbate 80 (P80)	↓ Diversity ↓ *Faecalibacterium, Bifidobacterium*	↓ Mucus layer thickness ↑ Permeability	↑ Intestinal inflammation	Crohn's disease Ulcerative colitis Colorectal cancer Type 1 diabetes Alzheimer's disease Obesity Colon cancer IBS
	Kappa carrageenan	↑ *E. coli, Shigella*	↑ LPS	↑ Intestinal inflammation	Crohn's disease Ulcerative colitis Diabetes Colon cancer IBS
Food colorants	Titanium dioxide nanoparticles	↓ Diversity ↑ Firmicutes ↓ *Lactobacillus, Bifidobacteria, Akkermansia* ↓ SCFAs	↑ Permeability	↑ Inflammation ↑ IL-23	Crohn's disease Ulcerative colitis Colon cancer IBS
	Red 40 (Allura red) Yellow 6 (Sunset yellow)	↓ Diversity with high-fat diet	ANSA-Na metabolites cross the gut barrier	↑ Intestinal inflammation ↑ IL-23	IBS Ulcerative colitis ADHD Allergic reactions

These are not just lab results. We have human studies in which we see that seven days of saccharin use alters blood sugar response and the gut microbiome in healthy humans. When the researchers did a fecal transplant from the people into mice, the mice developed altered blood sugar responses but were perfectly fine when they got a fecal transplant from the research participant *before* he or she started taking saccharin. Saccharin is found in common baked goods, jams and jelly, chewing gum, and salad dressings.

In a double-blind clinical trial, just eleven days of carboxymethyl-cellulose (CMC) exposure was enough to reduce gut diversity, allow microbial invasion of the mucus layer, and trigger gut symptoms in healthy individuals who didn't have these problems when they started. CMC is often found in ice cream, sweets, yogurt, and diet foods.

To be clear, the associations between food additives and human disease are not definitively "proven." True proof requires long-term human testing to capture the effect of chronic exposure, ideally as part of a randomized, controlled trial. But we can't get our regulators to mandate basic feeding studies, let alone rigorous human testing. Suffice it to say, gold standard research on food additives is never ever going to happen. But make no mistake. The big experiment is happening; it's just that we are the guinea pigs.

Meanwhile, autoimmune diseases continue to skyrocket as tens of thousands of untested additives enter our diets at varying times, in varying amounts, across diverse populations. Food labels rarely specify how much of these additives they contain—if they bother to list them at all—making it nearly impossible to identify a single culprit. More important, how do we account for the possibility that these illnesses stem from the combined effects of multiple substances interacting with a genetically predisposed individual rather than one clear-cut cause? These challenges arise because we introduce new additives under the assumption of safety, only to scramble for proof of harm afterward. Ultimately, all we can do is gather converging lines of evidence—from shifts in the microbiome to changes in the immune system to patterns of disease—that consistently point in the same worrisome direction.

What I come back to is this: If the three to five pounds of food that you eat per day are coming into contact with your gut bugs to produce short-chain fatty acids, neurotransmitters, hormones, vitamins, and other postbiotics that have the power to alter human physiology, tilting you toward health or disease, then it would seem that health and food are indeed inseparable. We are right to be concerned about untested and minimally labeled food additives.

A Horror Novel in One Paragraph. Eat Your Heart Out, Stephen King!

We're going to play a little game. I will list the ingredients in a commonly used product, and you will guess what it is as you read forward line by line. Here goes: nonfat milk, lactose, vegetable oil (palm olein, coconut, soy, and high oleic sunflower oils), whey protein concentrate, galactooligosaccharides, polydextrose, mortierella alpina oil, cryptocodinium cohnii oil, calcium carbonate, potassium citrate, ferrous sulfate, potassium chloride, magnesium oxide, sodium chloride, zinc sulfate, cupric sulfate, manganese sulfate, potassium iodide, sodium selenite, soy lecithin, choline chloride, ascorbic acid, niacinamide, calcium pantothenate, vitamin A palmitate, vitamin B_{12}, vitamin D_3, riboflavin, thiamin hydrochloride, vitamin B_6 hydrochloride, folic acid, vitamin K_1, biotin, inositol, vitamin E acetate, nucleotides (cytidine 5'-monophosphate, disodium uridine 5'-monophosphate, adenosine 5'-monophosphate, disodium guanosine 5'-monophosphate), taurine, l-carnitine. What is it? That is the number one selling infant formula in the United States. Need I say more? Nope.

Alcohol and the Microbiome:
The Study That Changed My Opinion

It's been clear for many years that heavy alcohol consumption has serious consequences: cirrhosis, alcoholic fatty liver, and alcoholic hepatitis, to name a few. These are all manifestations of the gut-liver axis—the two-way communication between the gut and liver, where gut microbes and gut barrier integrity influence liver health through immune signaling, toxins, and microbe-produced bioactives. But this connection works both ways—as alcohol use disorder progresses, it progressively damages the gut microbiome, further fueling liver dysfunction. It's the same destructive cycle—a broken microbiome leads to a weakened gut barrier, triggering inflammation that spreads from the gut to the liver, pushing the body further toward disease. But the damage doesn't stop at the liver. Chronic alcohol abuse also takes a toll on other organs, contributing to conditions like pancreatitis, gastritis, neuropathy, heart failure, depression, Alzheimer's disease, epilepsy, inflammatory bowel disease, microscopic colitis, psoriasis, type 2 diabetes, high blood pressure, coronary artery disease, stroke, fetal alcohol syndrome, and at least fourteen different types of cancer.

But there's a difference between abuse and use. We've been hearing for a long time that moderate alcohol consumption, defined as one drink per day for women and two for men, is actually good for us. This idea really coalesced after a 2011 systematic review and meta-analysis showing lower risk of death from cardiovascular disease among moderate drinkers. Red wine has even been associated with increased gut diversity, which is thought to be due to the polyphenol resveratrol. Beer has its own polyphenols that come from hops, and many believe they are beneficial to our gut bugs as well. So while I generally maintained that less is more and wrote in *Fiber Fueled* that "the safest amount of alcohol is none," I've had periods of time where I've indulged in a nightly glass of red wine. Did I do this 100 percent for the health benefits? No. I also did it because I enjoyed it.

But I changed my mind when I came across this study: Twenty-five healthy adults who were moderate or less drinkers were given enough alcohol to raise their blood alcohol level to 0.08 percent, which is the legal limit for driving throughout most of the United States. They then checked their blood every thirty minutes for four hours and again the following day. Here's what they found: Serum LPS (lipopolysaccharide) levels spiked immediately and remained elevated for three hours. Bacteria actually flooded into the bloodstream. They knew because they could detect a surge in bacterial DNA. Inflammatory cytokines shot up. In other words, the alcohol was punching holes in the gut barrier.

There are two things that were buried in the paper that really hit hardest for me. First, LPS levels rose and fell in parallel to blood alcohol levels. When alcohol goes up, so does LPS. When alcohol goes down, so does LPS. Second, the LPS level didn't return to normal until the alcohol level did. Collectively, this underscores just how closely linked our gut barrier is to alcohol levels.

My concern is that even minimal alcohol may damage the gut barrier. Recently, there have been challenges to the idea that moderate alcohol intake is actually good for us. New analyses show that the benefits of moderate alcohol disappear when one accounts for biases and confounders. Furthermore, even a single alcoholic drink is enough to disrupt sleep. Based upon this, if you have a chronic inflammatory condition, you're taking the chance that regular alcohol consumption is actually fueling your inflammatory fire.

My journey to kick alcohol is one of my many progress-over-perfection stories. Yes, I am an author, internationally recognized gastroenterologist, and health and wellness expert. But I'm 100 percent human and imperfect. Reducing my alcohol use isn't about being perfect. But it is about making choices in my life that are consistent with where the science leads me. I'll still enjoy a drink on occasion, provided it's being shared with a friend.

Should We Reach for the Wacky Tobacky Instead of the Booze?

Cannabis use is becoming more popular. People enjoy it, and I get it! But there are a number of disturbing possibilities associated with marijuana use. First, there are the cognitive effects. Long-term cannabis use is associated with cognitive loss, IQ decline, poor learning, and slower processing speed. We used to call this being a "pothead." Brain imaging of chronic marijuana users has shown shrinking of their hippocampus, the part of their brain associated with memory, learning, and emotion. Yes, I just said that. Their brains shrank.

Second, there are the gut effects. Chronic cannabis use is associated with cyclic vomiting syndrome and a condition called cannabinoid hyperemesis syndrome, something I've seen increasingly in recent years and particularly among young people. Here's how this plays out: They come to see me with chronic nausea and vomiting, and my first question is, "Do you love taking hot showers?" Their eyes bug out and they look at me like, "OMG, how did you know?" I wish I were telepathic, but I'm not. This is your gut on marijuana. First, chronic marijuana use causes morning nausea and abdominal discomfort. But paradoxically, marijuana use actually helps the nausea. So the user increases their marijuana use, trying to fix the problem. Then things get way, way, way worse. Eventually, the user develops cannabinoid hyperemesis syndrome, which can cause them to violently throw up for hours on end. Interestingly, there's one thing that helps them feel better—a hot shower. So they compulsively spend tons of time in the shower. The only way this goes away is to stop using weed permanently, which requires overcoming their physical and psychological dependence.

There's also the association of cannabis use with increased risk of car crashes, vision impairment, paranoia, depression, mania, and even psychosis. And so, the risks associated with marijuana use are not trivial. But there are also suggested benefits: Marijuana can reduce seizures in epilepsy, lessen spasticity in multiple sclerosis, improve quality of life for people with inflammatory bowel disease, and relieve the chronic pain associated with various conditions.

So where do I land on marijuana? It's possible that there's a form and amount of cannabis that's actually beneficial to our gut, gut barrier, and immune system. But we don't know what that is, and cannabis also comes with the risk of serious cognitive, gut, mood, and other adverse effects. I'm looking for more data, but until then I'm staying on the side of, "It's a no for me, dawg."

What About Tobacco or E-cigs?

We can keep this short and sweet: Yes, smoking negatively impacts your gut microbiome and gut barrier function, and it causes mass scale inflammation. By the way, e-cigarettes appear to do this as well, so you're not off the hook there. We all know that smoking is associated with multiple forms of cancer, heart disease, stroke, and chronic obstructive pulmonary disease. Those, unfortunately, are the OG outcomes of tobacco use. A new generation of smoking-related disorders is now emerging: Crohn's disease, rheumatoid arthritis, ankylosing spondylitis, spondyloarthritis, psoriasis and psoriatic arthritis, systemic and cutaneous lupus, multiple sclerosis, primary biliary cholangitis, Buerger's disease, and myasthenia gravis.

Let's Take It Home

The idea here is rather simple. What we consider normal in today's world is anything but normal when viewed through the lens of 99.9999 percent of human history. We've drastically altered our environment—and with it, the delicate ecosystem of our gut microbes. Like it or not, we are products of our environment, and the one we've created is dysbiotic on both a macro and micro level.

This chapter only scratches the surface. Our day-to-day challenges extend far beyond the food that we eat or the beverages we drink. It can feel quite overwhelming to consider the many toxic exposures we face daily, and there are other books that elaborate eloquently on all of the different possibilities that exist in our world. But here's the key takeaway—true health is absolutely possible in today's world. Science gives us the tools we need to heal our microbiome, gut barrier, and immune system. Rather than trying to find the solution in the past, I believe we have the opportunity to forge a new and better future—one shaped by an informed, modern approach to gut-immune health. That's the essence of *Plant Powered Plus*—the blueprint for thriving in a world full of challenges. In Part II, I'll show you exactly how we can do that. Flip the page. I'll meet you there.

Chapter 3 is backed by 428 references gathered through an extensive review of the scientific literature. You can browse the full citation list at www .theguthealthmd.com/plantpoweredplus.

THE PILLARS OF GUT-IMMUNE HEALTH

Strategies for Thriving in the Modern World

MAKING IT SUSTAINABLE

Plant Powered and Unrestricted

Across from me sat Candace, a patient I hadn't seen for a while. At fifty-two, she'd weathered the storm of ulcerative colitis and at our last visit had finally found a steady rhythm with her medication. At that time, her gut was calm and in a good place. But just when she thought she was back on track, another issue surfaced—joint pain. "Most of the time it's just a dull ache in my wrist or knee. I notice it, but it's not a huge deal. But occasionally one of them flares up—hot, swollen, tight, and very tender," she explained. Peripheral arthritis, joint pain in the arms and legs that often moves from one joint to another, can be an unwelcome companion to ulcerative colitis, a reminder that inflammation doesn't always confine itself to one area.

"I read about diets that might help and so far I've tried the specific carbohydrate diet (SCD) and the autoimmune protocol (AIP), but they were both so restrictive that I couldn't keep them up," she told me. "I read on a message board recently that people with inflammatory bowel diseases have a higher risk of heart disease. I love food. I want it to taste good. And I want relief from my arthritis now as well as something that will help my long-term health. Is that too much to ask?"

I know there are many of you out there like Candace who are trying to figure out what to eat to reduce inflammation and improve your health both now and in the future. The most popular diets in the last few years purporting to help with chronic inflammatory conditions have been variations on the low-carb diet. The specific carbohydrate diet was developed in 1920 to treat celiac disease, but it is seeing a resurgence among people with inflammatory bowel disease. The autoimmune protocol, an even more restrictive version of the Paleo diet, is trendy among people with autoimmune disease, particularly those with autoimmune thyroid disease. More recently there's been a surge in interest in the carnivore diet, which, as the name suggests, includes just meat or just animal-based foods.

If you've used these diets, were able to stick with them, and had success with them, I'm happy to hear it. Certainly, these diets will make you feel better in the short term if you're transitioning away from an inflammatory Western diet. Why? Because the thing they all have in common is the elimination of ultra-processed, ultra-refined foods. Each of these diets—SCD, AIP, and carnivore—is a structured approach to get more real food and less ultra-processed foods. I support that general concept. There's merit to prioritizing minimally processed whole foods.

But some things are good in the short term and bad in the long term—or come with compromises in other areas of your health. The problem is that these diets also ask you to eliminate healthful foods. The SCD diet, for example, eliminates all hard-to-digest carbohydrates, effectively restricting complex carbs like whole grains, legumes, and starchy vegetables. The AIP diet goes even further, cutting out entire categories of plant foods, including whole grains, legumes, nuts, seeds, and nightshade vegetables. The carnivore diet takes this to the extreme, eliminating every single plant food—fruits, vegetables, whole grains, nuts, seeds, and legumes. Do you see a pattern emerging?

These diets systematically remove plant-based foods that are rich in prebiotics—the very compounds that feed the good bacteria in your gut. Fewer prebiotics means fewer short-chain fatty acids (SCFAs), the critical anti-inflammatory compounds that support your gut microbes, strengthen your gut barrier, and regulate your immune system. As we learned in Chapter 1, SCFAs are essential for the symbiotic growth of all three systems, allowing them to thrive together. So here's the paradox: We need a healthy gut to support a healthy immune system, yet we're tackling chronic inflammatory conditions by cutting out the very foods that make our gut healthier. Does that make sense?

We could do worse (see Chapter 3), but I also think we can do better—much better. Are these plant foods really the root cause of our modern epidemics? It seems unlikely when people are eating less of them now than at any other time in human history. Every plant food contains dietary fiber, yet 90 percent of women and 97 percent of men are fiber deficient. Shockingly, the percentage of Americans consuming the recommended daily servings of these foods is alarmingly low: fruits, 20 percent; legumes, 15 percent; vegetables, 10 percent; and whole grains, a pathetic 2 percent. Meanwhile, overwhelming evidence supports the benefits of fiber-rich plant foods for human health on so many different levels. Sorry, but I don't believe the foods that we're deficient in are the cause of our epidemics or our inflammation. The restrictive diets have gone too far. We're throwing the baby out with the bathwater.

There are no long-term studies on the SCD, AIP, or carnivore diets. The SCD and AIP each have a tiny little morsel of evidence to suggest benefit for celiac disease and thyroid disease, respectively. It's not enough, but in a world that's devoid of nutritional research, it is worth acknowledging. The carnivore diet is a zero fiber diet. You'd have to completely ignore the thousands of studies that demonstrate tremendous health benefits of fiber to the gut, to the immune system, and to human health in general in order to believe in this approach. There's actually only one study to support the carnivore diet, and it's honestly the most poorly conducted study that I'm citing in this entire book. In it, they used social media to find 2,029 people who were actively doing a carnivore diet for six months or more and asked them about their experience. Unsurprisingly, when you survey an online echo chamber devoted to a diet, you're going to get glowing reviews—it's like asking the Taylor Swift fan club if she deserves another Grammy. To their credit, the study did acknowledge one glaring issue—participants had severely elevated LDL cholesterol, the "bad" cholesterol linked to cardiovascular disease. No surprise there—this is exactly what happens when you load up on saturated fat while cutting out fiber entirely. Thankfully, Dr. Alan Flanagan wrote a letter to the editor to highlight some of the issues with both the study and an exclusively animal-based approach. Ultra-restrictive low-carb diets that increase our saturated fat and salt intake while depriving us of fiber, magnesium, potassium, and vitamins A, E, D, C, and folate are far from balanced, suffering from the massive excesses of animal-based foods and exposing us to serious nutritional deficiencies due to the absence of plant-based foods.

I'm going to tell you what I told Candace that day: I don't want you on a wildly restrictive diet that cuts out the foods that we know are essential for long-term gut health and longevity. Your gut health is far too precious—it's the foundation for a strong gut barrier and a well-functioning immune system. While it's tempting to avoid certain foods to minimize symptoms, I want more for you than short-term relief with long-term consequences. We want to heal your microbiome. My goal is to guide you toward a dietary pattern that nurtures your microbes, repairs your gut barrier, and reduces inflammation. And I'll help you make it your own so that it tastes good, doesn't feel restrictive, and can become a foundation of health for the rest of your life. There's no one-size-fits-all when it comes to diet. Everyone's body responds differently, and what works wonders for one person might not be the answer for another. Instead of trying to force a rigid plan on you, let's get the fundamentals in place and let you choose your own delicious adventure.

The foundational foods we will talk about in this chapter are what the healthiest people on the planet eat. They promote longevity by consistently reducing inflammation. They are grounded in rock-solid science. And, they are foods that have always been a part of our biology through our evolutionary history. It's time for us to reconnect with this way of eating. I call it getting Plant Powered.

Getting Plant Powered

I've been around long enough to see that all kinds of diets can help people thrive, and there's no universal standard solution. At the same time, my approach isn't "Eat what you want, anything goes." Our goal is to reduce inflammation and help you live longer, healthier, and with more vitality by nurturing your microbiome and repairing and restoring the gut barrier. That's what being Plant Powered is about. So how do we get there? First, we're going to lean on published research—using the best data available to guide our choices. Second, we'll look to real-world examples, not cave dwellers who had no cars, no air-conditioning, and no idea what a smartphone was. They may share your biology, but they don't share your environment. Instead, let's explore modern cultures around the globe where people are thriving and see what we can learn from their eating habits and lifestyles. Together, we'll identify the core tenets of a diet that meets our goals: flexible, science-backed, decidedly not restrictive, and yes—absolutely delicious.

A Plant Powered diet simply means: whole, fiber-rich plants front and center, with flexibility for your tastes. Think of it as a spectrum—not a straitjacket—so you can begin where you are, progress at your own pace, and build a pattern that's both joyful and health-promoting.

But Wait, Doc, I Thought I Was Supposed to Go Plant-Based?

You absolutely are. But let's start by defining what that means. Eating plant-based isn't about a rigid label—it's about prioritizing plants for health while acknowledging the overwhelming evidence that people thrive when they eat more fiber-rich, nutrient-dense plant foods. This isn't all-or-nothing; it's about progress. In *Plant Powered Plus*, the focus is on making the healthiest choices for your body, reducing inflammation, and fueling your gut microbiome.

That being said, health motivations are different from ethical motivations. I respect and admire those who align their diet with their values. We all should strive to do that. But here, we're focused on personalizing nutrition—finding the optimal anti-inflammatory diet that works for you.

To accomplish this, I want to meet you where you are. If I can help you move from 10 percent to 30 percent plant-based, that's progress, and I celebrate that. But I'd love to see you continue—from 50 percent to 70 percent—progressing until one day you are 90 percent or more plant-based. That's the long-term goal. But I also know firsthand that it's a journey—one that took me years to navigate myself. This isn't about shame, guilt, or pressure (which, by the way, only makes gut issues worse—see Chapter 8). Instead, I want you to understand that healing takes time—it's a slightly different process for each of us—and to know that I support you.

If you have serious health issues, you are starting with deeper dysbiosis and will require more time for healing. A plants-only approach may not be possible now, or even for a while. That's okay. In *Plant Powered Plus*, we take a gradual, adaptive approach, allowing time for your gut to adjust and for you to meet your nutritional needs—even if that means incorporating some animal-based foods along the way. Over time, there will be opportunities to add more plants, and patience and persistence will be key.

Sustainability is everything. If including some animal-based foods helps you feel your best, I want to be the one who supports you in finding that balance—one that keeps plants at the center while respecting what works for your body. At the end of the day, my goal isn't to push a rigid ideology—it's to help guide you toward a superior diet. That generally means more plants, healthier fats, and, for some of you, some thoughtfully chosen animal-based foods.

A Mediterranean Approach: Ancient Traditions and a Culinary Crossroads

In the early 1950s, American scientist Ancel Keys wanted to understand the rise of heart disease, which had taken over as the top cause of death. He brought together a team of research collaborators from across the globe—the United States, Japan, the Netherlands, Finland, Yugoslavia, Italy, and Greece—and together they started what's called the Seven Countries Study.

As the results came in, Ancel was struck by a discovery that seemed paradoxical and surprising. Poor people living in small towns in southern Italy were much healthier than wealthy citizens of New York. He described the Italians' diet as "lots of fresh vegetables sprinkled with olive oil, a small portion of meat or fish maybe a couple of times a week, and always fresh fruit for dessert" and showed how this simple, plant-forward way of eating correlated strongly with a lower risk of heart disease.

This was the very beginning of nutritional epidemiology and unlocking our understanding of how our food choices can inform our health. Amazingly, what was discovered in the 1950s has since been studied extensively and matured far beyond heart health to become a modern microbiome-nurturing, gut-barrier-restoring, immune-supporting diet.

The Mediterranean Diet

In recent years, I've been the US Medical Director of a personalized nutrition company called ZOE and served on their scientific advisory board. ZOE runs the world's largest, most in-depth nutritional research program, focused on uncovering how each of us uniquely interacts with food—and how we can make healthier choices as a result. While this research informs ZOE's membership program, it also gets published in top scientific journals so that many more will benefit. Our mission is to improve the health of millions.

The ZOE PREDICT study involved 1,098 people (including 480 twins!) who did microbiome testing and extensive biomarker testing, and wore a continuous blood sugar monitor for two weeks. It was game-changing for understanding how food influences our microbes and our health and produced multiple papers published in *Nature Medicine*, the top medical journal on the planet. In one of these breakthrough papers, ZOE researchers identified fifteen "good" and fifteen "bad" gut bugs that were connected to important facets of human health—inflammation; blood sugar and blood fat responses to food; and cardiovascular risk. Together we call them the ZOE Microbiome Score. Increase your good gut bugs and diminish your bad gut bugs and you tilt the scale in the favor of your health.

The Mediterranean diet showed up loud and clear in the gut microbiome—so much so that researchers could tell if someone was following this eating pattern just by analyzing their microbes. Of all the diets studied, it correlated most strongly with the thirty gut bugs that make up the ZOE Microbiome Score. Specifically, people who closely followed a Mediterranean-style diet significantly boosted eleven of the fifteen "good" microbes while suppressing fourteen of the fifteen "bad" ones. In other words, by embracing a Mediterranean approach, you're actively fine-tuning the most critical players in your gut toward better health.

A Mediterranean diet isn't just a delicious way to eat—it's a powerhouse for your gut. Studies have consistently shown that this way of eating is associated with a more diverse microbiome, which is a key marker of gut health. In fact, one small interventional study found that just two weeks on a Mediterranean diet was enough to increase gut diversity, and that's not too shabby for a mere fortnight of change. But the benefits don't stop at microbial variety. Those who closely follow a Mediterranean diet also exhibit higher levels of short-chain fatty acids, crucial compounds that repair and maintain our gut barrier, along with lower levels of harmful substances like TMAO (trimethylamine N-oxide). This connection was confirmed in a randomized controlled trial where women with damaged gut barriers adopted a Mediterranean diet. After just three months, their short-chain fatty acid levels had risen significantly and their gut barriers were notably repaired. As I've often said, short-chain fatty acids are powerfully anti-inflammatory, underscoring how a Mediterranean approach not only enriches our microbiome but also fortifies the very barriers that protect our immune system.

This anti-inflammatory effect is measurable and significant. Seven different markers of inflammation drop lower on a Mediterranean diet—CRP, IL-6, IL-8, TNF-α, IL-1β, E-selectin, and IFN-γ. Notably, the diet lowered TNF-α, which is important because it's the target of at least five different drugs called anti-TNFs that are used to treat ulcerative colitis, Crohn's disease, rheumatoid arthritis, psoriasis, psoriatic arthritis, and several other autoimmune conditions. Those drugs target one inflammatory cytokine, whereas our diet can target many.

With this in mind, you shouldn't be surprised that the Mediterranean diet can protect us from multiple autoimmune diseases: Crohn's disease, ulcerative colitis, rheumatoid arthritis, psoriatic arthritis, psoriasis, multiple sclerosis, Sjögren's, Hashimoto's disease, systemic

sclerosis, and fibromyalgia have all shown benefits from this diet.
What defines the Mediterranean dietary pattern? At its core, it's Plant
Powered—emphasizing a rainbow of colorful fruits and vegetables rich
in polyphenols and a variety of spices packed with anti-inflammatory
phytochemicals. At the same time, it requires you to improve the quality of the protein and fat in your diet. Combine these elements, and you
have a truly powerhouse anti-inflammatory diet.

Mediterranean Essentials

Colorful Vegetables & Fruits	At every meal
Whole Grains & Legumes	At every meal
Nuts & Seeds	At every meal
Herbs & Spices	At every meal
Extra-Virgin Olive Oil	At every meal

Weekly Additions

Fish, Shellfish & Bivalves	At least twice a week
Fermented Dairy (Yogurt, Kefir)	In moderation; limit unfermented dairy
Eggs & Poultry	In moderate amounts and small portions
Red Meat, Sweets	Rarely and small portions
Ultra-Processed Foods	Keep to a minimum

These are the core principles, but what's striking is that within
the history of Mediterranean food traditions, there's an extraordinary
amount of variation. In other words, there's no one rigid way to be
Plant Powered. The Mediterranean region has been called "the cradle of
society." It is home to Egypt and the pyramids, the Holy Land for three
major religions, and too many cultures and empires to count. It is also
the geographic crossroads between continents, where East meets West.

This region is a multi-millennial cultural melting pot, bringing to-gether the best and most delicious foods from a diverse mix of people.

Dating back to the first millennium CE, the Roman diet empha-sized bread, wine, and oil (central elements of the Christian liturgy) with olives, leeks, mushrooms, and other vegetables and a strong pref-erence for fish and seafood. The rich classes particularly loved oysters, either raw or fried in olive oil. The poor ate a diet heavy in bread, olives, olive oil, and salted fish. During the Early Middle ages, Germanic peo-ple lived in close harmony with the forest, growing vegetables in small gardens close to their camps. Islamic culture introduced lemons, al-monds, eggplant, spinach, and spices. And later on, the discovery of the New World in America introduced new foods, such as potatoes, toma-toes, corn, peppers, and a variety of beans.

Yes, we are talking about multiple different diets from different cul-tures, with culturally distinct food traditions. There's no one diet that serves them all. But they are connected by the foundational Plant Pow-ered principles of nutrition that are now highly researched and well documented. And this lesson informs our approach in this book: Once you have the building blocks, there are many different ways to be Plant Powered.

The Mediterranean Diet for Crohn's Disease and Ulcerative Colitis

Perhaps I'm biased because I'm a gastroenterologist, but to me these are the classic gut-immune diseases. All patients with inflam-matory bowel disease have dysbiosis and a damaged gut barrier. Their immune system reacts to this not by attacking itself (which would be autoimmune) but instead by attacking the gut microbiome, which it has determined is the enemy. The result is massive, debili-tating inflammation in the intestines and, in some cases, outside the intestines.

In a study, patients with Crohn's disease and ulcerative colitis followed the Mediterranean diet for six months. What happened? They were less likely to have active disease or high inflammation in their blood work. They improved their quality of life. They also lost weight, shrank their waist circumference, and reduced their liver fat—meaning they were metabolically healthier in addition to being less inflamed. This study exemplifies why recently updated gastro-enterology guidelines in inflammatory bowel disease state, "Unless there is a contraindication, all patients with IBD should be advised to follow a Mediterranean diet." Mic drop.

We Were Told to Go "Low-Fat," and Then Along Came Research

In the late twentieth century, dietary fat became the villain of our plates. Grocery aisles transformed into battlegrounds lined with "low-fat" and "fat-free" products, all promising better health and slimmer waistlines. The prevailing wisdom was simple: Fat was the enemy, clogging our arteries and expanding our waistlines. Health authorities, nutritionists, and doctors rallied behind this message, urging everyone to cut fat wherever possible.

Yet, amid this crusade against fat, a curious paradox emerged from the sun-drenched coasts of the Mediterranean. In countries like Italy, Greece, and Spain, people were drizzling olive oil over their salads, enjoying handfuls of nuts and fatty fish. Their diets were inherently high in fat—precisely what we were told to avoid. But instead of suffering from rampant heart disease, these populations exhibited some of the lowest rates of cardiovascular issues globally. Study after study from Denmark to the United States confirmed the protective benefits of the Mediterranean diet.

This contradiction couldn't be ignored. Intrigued by these findings, a team of dedicated researchers in Spain decided to dive deeper. Funded by their government, they initiated the PREDIMED study—a landmark trial designed to compare the high-fat Mediterranean diet directly against a traditional low-fat diet. Their goal was to challenge the entrenched beliefs about dietary fat and provide concrete evidence on how these diets impacted heart health.

To accomplish this, they recruited 7,447 individuals aged fifty-five to eighty who had either type 2 diabetes or multiple cardiovascular risk factors—like smoking, being overweight, high blood pressure, abnormal blood lipids, or a family history of heart disease—but none had experienced a heart attack or stroke themselves. In other words, these were people at great risk for cardiovascular disease. From 2003 to 2011, across eleven teaching hospitals, these participants were followed for an average of five years. They were randomly assigned to one of three diets: a Mediterranean diet supplemented with 4 tablespoons of extra-virgin olive oil per day, a Mediterranean diet supplemented with 30 grams of mixed nuts per day, or a low-fat diet. There were no calorie restrictions; participants could eat as much or as little as they wanted. So to summarize: 7,500 people, eleven medical centers, three diets, five years = one ROCKSTAR study that was a modern nutrition game changer.

The findings from the PREDIMED study painted a vivid picture of the Mediterranean diet's profound impact on health compared to that of a low-fat diet. Participants who followed the Mediterranean diets, whether supplemented with EVOO or nuts, experienced a significant reduction in heart attacks, strokes, and death from cardiovascular causes compared to those who were on the low-fat diet. The Mediterranean diet literally gave them a second chance at life.

We see this on a biochemical level. Participants saw their levels of LDL cholesterol, often dubbed the "bad" cholesterol, drop lower, and their blood pressure readings improved, both critical factors in cardiovascular health. Heart failure biomarkers improved, suggesting better overall heart function. Cognition also improved, suggesting benefits that extend to brain health. This could have meaningful implications for aging populations concerned about memory and cognitive decline.

But perhaps most striking were the reductions in inflammatory markers. Inflammation is a key player in many chronic diseases, and the Mediterranean diet seems to tackle it head-on. Participants exhibited lower levels of inflammatory markers related to atherosclerosis. Specifically, C-reactive protein (CRP) levels were 35 to 45 percent less, and interleukin-6 (IL-6) levels were 90 to 95 percent less compared to a low-fat diet. Such substantial decreases highlight the diet's potent anti-inflammatory effects.

Keep in mind that not all fats are created equal. The Mediterranean diet specifically pushes you to prioritize the higher-quality fats—EVOO, nuts and seeds, seafood—and to limit sources of saturated fat. Instead of fearing fat, it's about embracing the right kinds—those that nourish the body and support overall health.

The Role of EVOO in a Mediterranean Diet

Perhaps you noticed that extra-virgin olive oil, or EVOO, is a big part of the Mediterranean diet. And this may seem confusing because there are some experts who are highly intelligent and well educated who believe that we are healthiest when we are oil-free. Many of them are my friends whom I respect and cherish.

In the PREDIMED study, the EVOO group was kicking back 4 tablespoons of EVOO *daily*. That's not a small amount! That's about 480 calories per day from EVOO alone. And remember, calories weren't being restricted, so this was something that they added to everything else they were eating.

The fascinating part is that they did INCREDIBLY well, with a litany of benefits that people on a Mediterranean diet experienced whether including EVOO or nuts. But there were some health benefits experienced only by those on the EVOO-supplemented diet, including lower rates of breast cancer, lower rates of type 2 diabetes, lower rates of diabetic retinopathy, lower rates of non-alcoholic fatty liver disease, and lower rates of atrial fibrillation when compared to those following the low-fat diet.

My take: There are many paths to health, and you need to find what works for you. You can absolutely be healthy and be oil-free if that's what you prefer. But I've just shown you evidence that people can be healthy with EVOO. The principle is simple: When you add EVOO, you are adding high-quality fat to your diet. One caveat, though—an extra 480 calories per day with zero fiber isn't ideal, even if it's from EVOO, if you are obese or trying to lose weight.

From Loma Linda with Love

Dan Buettner is no ordinary researcher—he's a modern-day explorer and National Geographic Fellow who has turned the quest for longevity into a thrilling adventure. In the early 2000s, armed with a deep curiosity and a passion for uncovering life's greatest secrets, Dan set out to identify the pockets of the world where people were not just living longer but thriving well into their centenarian years.

Dan's work as a National Geographic Fellow wasn't confined to laboratories or libraries; it took him across continents and into the heart of communities untouched by the frenetic pace of modern life. Yes, he found places with thriving humans who were living to be one hundred years old at a rate that was off the charts. But beyond the data, what he really found were authentic stories of the human experience—vivid tapestries of lives filled with purpose, connection, and health.

Using a simple blue marker on an old-fashioned map, Dan circled these extraordinary regions, five of them, and thus the term "Blue Zones," geographic regions where people live longer and healthier lives than average, was born. Two of the five Blue Zones are Mediterranean— Icaria and Sardinia. But one of these locations isn't tucked away in a remote mountain village or an isolated island, and it's got a unique dietary pattern that has a lot to tell us about the power of flexible Plant Powered diets—it's right here in the United States, in Loma Linda, California. Dan described this city as a "longevity oasis," where residents live up to a decade longer than the average American. What was their secret?

Roughly half of Loma Linda's population belongs to the Seventh-day Adventist Church, a Protestant Christian denomination that views health as a spiritual practice. Adventists believe that their bodies are temples of the Holy Spirit—a gift to be cared for with intention and respect. This philosophy permeates every aspect of their lives, from the food they eat to the way they interact with their community.

Intrigued by the remarkable health and longevity of this group, researchers initiated the Adventist Health Study-2 in 2002. This extensive study followed 96,194 Adventists across North America to explore the connections between their dietary habits and disease risk. The results were nothing short of astounding. Adventist women were found to live 4.4 years longer and Adventist men 7.3 years longer than other Californians. They experienced lower rates of heart disease, diabetes, and certain cancers.

The best way to describe the general diet of the Adventists is Plant Powered. Around half of the Adventists follow a vegetarian, vegan, pescatarian, or flexitarian diet, emphasizing whole, plant-based foods rich in fiber, antioxidants, and essential nutrients. These foods not only nourish the body but also support a healthy gut microbiome and reduce systemic inflammation.

The Adventist community offers a unique opportunity to study these less common, Plant Powered dietary patterns. Although chronic inflammatory and autoimmune conditions are not the focus of the Adventist-2 study, there have been several notable discoveries. A vegan diet may be associated with lower risk of hypothyroid disease. Vegan, vegetarian, and pescatarian diets may protect against hyperthyroidism. And there were lower rates of lupus among those who follow a vegetarian or pescatarian diet.

What the study did focus on was metabolic health conditions associated with chronic inflammation, including heart disease, stroke, diabetes, and obesity. If you looked below the hood at someone with any of these conditions, or the precursors to these conditions, you would find a diseased microbiome and a damaged gut barrier. What did the Adventist Health Study-2 show in regard to vegetarian, vegan, pescatarian, or flexitarian diets and these conditions?

For those embracing a vegan lifestyle, the benefits were striking. Compared to their omnivorous counterparts, vegans were:

- **16 percent less likely to be diagnosed with cancer.** This suggests that a plant-exclusive diet may offer protective effects against cancer development.

- **63 percent less likely to be diagnosed with high blood pressure.** High blood pressure is a major risk factor for heart disease and stroke, so this reduction is significant.

- **62 percent less likely to be diagnosed with type 2 diabetes.** Given the global rise of diabetes, this is a powerful testament to the impact of dietary choices.

Vegetarians, who include dairy and eggs in their plant-based diet, also saw considerable health advantages:

- **43 percent less likely to be diagnosed with high blood pressure.**

- **38 percent less likely to be diagnosed with type 2 diabetes.**

Pescatarians, those who add fish to a vegetarian diet, emerged as the longevity champions in the study:

- **19 percent less likely to die during the study period.** In fact, pescatarians were the longest-lived participants in the study.

- **35 percent less likely to die from a heart attack.** We'll discuss omega-3s in the next chapter, but bookmark this in your mind.

- **42 percent less likely to be diagnosed with colorectal cancer.** This is noteworthy, as colorectal cancer is the second leading cause of cancer death in America.

Even those who identified as **semi-vegetarian or flexitarian,** eating mostly plants but incorporating meat occasionally, experienced benefits:

- **51 percent less likely to be diagnosed with type 2 diabetes.**

The study also revealed a clear progression in body mass index (BMI), a key indicator of healthy weight, based on dietary choices:

	VEGAN	VEGETARIAN	PESCATARIAN	FLEXITARIAN	OMNIVORE
BMI	24.0	25.9	26.2	27.2	28.6

There are various dietary paths, but they all emphasize increased plant consumption and share a common thread of providing significant advantages—not only in immediate reductions in inflammation markers but also in long-term health outcomes. These progressive improvements in BMI highlight the power of plant-based diets to combat obesity, enhance metabolic health, extend longevity, and lower systemic inflammation. By embracing a lifestyle centered on plant foods, we pave the way for a future of sustained vitality and reduced risk of chronic disease.

Put simply, when you add more plants to your plate, you are moving in the right direction. Embracing a simple way of life that honors our bodies and fills our plates with nourishing plant-based foods is good for your gut, and it's also good for your longevity and long-term health. This is the Plant Powered way. Let's not also miss that in Loma Linda, they are strongly connected to one another through meaningful relationships, and their faith gives them a strong sense of purpose. This is being Plant Powered Plus. We'll come back to these concepts in Chapter 8.

What's a Flexitarian?

	VEGAN	VEGETARIAN	PESCATARIAN	FLEXITARIAN (SEMI-VEGETARIAN)
Meat	None	None	None	Very little
Fish	None	None	Included	Included
Eggs	None	Included (if ovovegetarian)	Optional	Included
Dairy	None	Included (if lactovegetarian)	Optional	Included
Vegetables	Lots	Lots	Lots	Lots
Fruits	Lots	Lots	Lots	Lots
Ultra-Processed Foods	Optional	Optional	Optional	Optional

Plant Powered in the Land of the Rising Sun

Japan is an island nation—a sprawling archipelago in the Pacific Ocean—where miles of coastline and centuries of cultural exchange have forged a distinctive way of life. Historically, the Japanese diet leaned heavily on fresh, seasonal foods from both land and sea. Vegetables, grains, legumes, seafood, and a range of fermented staples have long formed the culinary backbone of a diet that's whole food–based and rich in variety. This cultural framework, much like the Adventist community in Loma Linda, created a setting where a healthy diet and lifestyle were interwoven into daily life—not as a fleeting trend, but as a pillar of their cultural identity.

One of Dan Buettner's five Blue Zones, in fact, lies in Okinawa, a Japanese island known for its high concentration of centenarians. For generations, the people of Okinawa lived simply, ate locally, and cultivated tight-knit communities that supported them through life's challenges. Their dietary patterns were largely Plant Powered—fruits, vegetables, grains, legumes, and moderate amounts of fish—an approach that, like the Adventists', delivered longevity and robust health.

Yet as the tide of Westernization washed ashore in Japan, processed and ultra-processed foods—heavy on added sugars, refined flours, and industrial oils—have grown more common, particularly among younger generations. With this dietary shift has come a rise in health challenges that were once rare, including chronic inflammatory bowel diseases like Crohn's disease and ulcerative colitis.

For people with severe inflammatory bowel disease, there is a high level of intensity to their disease. They live every minute with a reminder of the fragility of their health, manifested with explosive diarrhea, blood in the stool, abdominal pain, and difficulty tolerating food. There is absolutely no doubt that medication is necessary in this setting. The health care system in the United States will happily provide this medicine, but it ignores the potential opportunity that exists when diet is combined with medicine.

Enter a group of innovative Japanese gastroenterologists who recognized this pattern and decided to push back. They suspected that the infiltration of Western dietary elements was altering the gut microbiome, replacing fiber-rich, whole-plant foods with ultra-processed and ultra-refined ones, and that this dietary shift was fueling the fires of inflammation. As early as 2003, these forward-thinking doctors set out to restore balance using a two-pronged approach for people with Crohn's disease and ulcerative colitis: medication plus a deliberate return to more traditional, plant-centric eating.

Patients were prescribed infliximab, a powerful anti-TNF medication that's used to treat both Crohn's disease and ulcerative colitis. This is a great medicine that I've had incredible success with through the years. But here's the twist: Instead of sticking to a standard Western diet, the patients were encouraged to adopt a semi-vegetarian pattern at the same time that they were starting their new medicine. They would eat mostly plants, incorporate fish on a weekly basis, and limit meat to roughly once every two weeks. This was no accident—it was designed to mirror the kinds of diets that generations of Japanese people had thrived on before Westernization took hold. In essence, it was a high-fiber, Plant Powered way of eating that would work in tandem with the medication.

You may recall our forest analogy from Chapter 2, where your microbiome is the forest, and inflammatory bowel disease is like a raging forest fire. In this study, the medicine is the fire hose putting out the fire, while the diet is planting the seeds to regrow the forest. They are not the same, but the combination is the optimal way to restore a lush, biodiverse forest.

The results were nothing short of remarkable. Of those with Crohn's disease who followed the combined approach—medicine plus the semi-vegetarian diet—96 percent achieved remission, meaning their disease essentially went quiet to the point that they couldn't feel it anymore. For comparison, remission rates hovered around 59 percent for those who took infliximab without changing their diet. Those results for infliximab are wonderful: Crohn's disease is a complex and difficult condition. But there's a big difference between twelve in twenty being better (with medicine alone) versus nineteen in twenty being better (with medicine *and* diet). Even more astonishing, more than half of the Crohn's disease patients who added diet to their medicine remained in remission for an entire decade, never once experiencing another flare-up. Read that again, because it's powerful. These patients started with a debilitating inflammatory disease, and they put it so deep into remission that they didn't have a flare-up for more than ten years. That's incredible.

Such success was not limited to Crohn's disease. Similar improvements were observed in those with severe ulcerative colitis. Markers of inflammation plummeted, surgical interventions dropped dramatically, and health outcomes improved. The C-reactive protein, a measure of inflammation throughout the body, dropped from 9.42, which is very high, to 0.33, which is very normal and not high at all.

These findings mirror what we learned from the Mediterranean diet and the flexitarian approach in Loma Linda: Plant Powered dietary patterns can reshape our internal environment, soothe the fires of inflammation, and restore health. Except here the research was most explicitly centered on taming an otherwise stubborn and debilitating inflammatory condition.

What does this mean for the rest of us? It suggests that the principles of a Plant Powered diet—deeply rooted in diverse whole plant foods—can serve as a powerful tool across cultures, continents, and conditions. We see it improve heart health. We see it promote longevity. We see it improve gut microbiome diversity. We have seen it turn the tide on Crohn's disease and ulcerative colitis. We've also seen that it's a diet with lots of room for flexibility and personal preference as well as plenty of delicious options. And in the broader context of our modern world, it shows us that we hold tremendous power on our plates.

Vegan Does Not Always Mean Whole Food and Plant-Based

The words "vegan" and "plant-based" are often conflated when they are not the same. Veganism is an ethical stance, fundamentally about refraining from consuming and wearing animal products to address concerns such as animal welfare and environmental impact. These issues are real and deserve our attention, but they are not automatically aligned with achieving better health. If a person goes vegan and replaces meat with soda, fries, and doughnuts, they have achieved their ethical goal but may not gain the health advantages we saw in Loma Linda's Adventist community.

A plant-based diet, on the other hand, is motivated by health. It's about emphasizing whole, minimally processed plant foods—fruits, vegetables, whole grains, legumes, nuts, and seeds—and reducing or eliminating animal products as a tool for better health outcomes. This includes a wide spectrum of dietary patterns that are all Plant Powered: whole food vegan, whole food vegetarian, pescatarian, flexitarian, and Mediterranean. They share a common foundation of starting with mostly plants, which is the key when moving toward an anti-inflammatory diet. Yet, at the same time, it's important to acknowledge that there are options, and each of us gets to choose what works best for us individually.

The distinction between vegan and whole foods plant-based diets is illustrated in a study from the United Kingdom called EPIC-Oxford. Researchers recruited over sixty-five thousand adults with a mix of dietary patterns. In contrast to the Adventist-2 study, which linked vegetarian and vegan diets to impressive longevity and health benefits, EPIC-Oxford's vegans and vegetarians didn't follow the same pattern. If you were to describe the groups in order from longest lived to shortest lived, it would go like this: semi-vegetarian (longest lived); pescatarian; vegetarian; vegan (least long lived). The differences between the groups were relatively small and not statistically significant, but nonetheless this is how the numbers shook out. Additionally, vegans and vegetarians had a higher risk of stroke. Now, don't get me wrong. The vegans and vegetarians weren't categorically less healthy. They had lower risk of heart disease, cancer, and diabetes, among others. But based upon everything we've discussed thus far, these results feel counterintuitive: How could people eating fewer animal products end up with worse outcomes?

The answer lies not in the simple absence of meat, but instead in what fills the plate (and the cup). Removal of meat doesn't necessarily result in more plants. In EPIC-Oxford, vegans and vegetarians consumed more sugar-sweetened beverages than pescatarians or omnivores. This isn't to blame soda consumption for the health differences. Instead, the soda intake is more a marker of an ultra-processed, ultra-refined diet. In EPIC-Oxford, the semi-vegetarians and pescatarians are eating for better health, while in general the vegans and vegetarians seem to be oriented toward their ethical motivations. Those are different goals, so it's not a surprise that they yield different results. Ultra-processed foods undermine the benefits of eating plants. Regardless of whether you're vegan, vegetarian, or omnivorous, junk food levels the playing field in a not-so-healthy way.

This is crucial because we are all on a journey. The way you eat today may be different from how you'll eat next year, and that's okay. My goal isn't to moralize or insist on a single rigid template. It's to guide you toward better health by leaning into the power of plants while acknowledging that there's room for individuality, personal growth, and gradual change. Some of you may start by simply adding a few more servings of vegetables in a smoothie or swapping out a soda for iced tea. This is how I started. Others might feel called to go entirely whole food, plant-exclusive. Both paths are valid, as is everything in between. Many paths can work. The key is quality and consistency over time.

A Word of Warning About Health Washing in Your Supermarket

Surely you've seen the terms "plant-based" and "non-GMO" plastered across food packaging. Perhaps more recently you've seen "prebiotic," and soon you'll see "postbiotic." These words in the right context indicate healthy choices, and food companies know this and are going to use that against you to market and sell their ultra-processed products. Make no mistake: An ultra-processed food labeled "plant-based" is still a UPF. Most snacks and beverages that claim "prebiotic" have added the cheapest, most-gas-producing fiber supplement to the UPF so that they can claim it's good for your gut. Don't fall for the trap! Here's a simple rule: Check the ingredients list. The longer it is, the more ultra-processed the product. If you can't pronounce half the ingredients, put it back. Buy real food whenever possible, and when you don't, choose options with the shortest, simplest ingredients list possible with ingredients that you actually recognize.

Plant Powered in Action

When Candace returned to my clinic several months later, she told me how she'd decided to build her own personal Plant Powered way of eating that suited both her taste buds and her health goals. She included Mediterranean elements, drawn to the olive oil, nuts, fruits, vegetables, and legumes, but she didn't feel boxed in. She allowed herself the flexibility to enjoy her favorite flavors, adding occasional fish or a sprinkle of cheese now and then. It wasn't about rigid rules but rather about elevating plants to the center of her plate and feeling good about it—not just physically but emotionally, too.

By centering her meals around whole, plant-based foods rich in antioxidants, fiber, and healthy fats, she naturally calmed her immune system, reduced systemic inflammation, and provided her joints with the nourishment they needed. Over time, she reported fewer bouts of joint pain, improved energy, and a sense of control over her own health destiny. As her body allowed, she slowly increased the amount of plant-based foods in her diet, and it worked incredibly well for her. She could literally feel how her dietary choices had a direct influence on her body's inflammatory state. Candace's journey illuminates the transformative power of a Plant Powered diet on inflammation.

Throughout this chapter, we've explored how different paths can lead to vibrant health and highlighted the flexibility and personalization that make dietary change sustainable. Yet clear patterns emerge— core nutritional pillars consistently linked to reduced inflammation and thriving gut health. What exactly are these foundational elements at the heart of every healthful Plant Powered diet? I'm going to show you in Chapter 5.

Chapter 4 is backed by 87 references gathered through an extensive review of the scientific literature. You can browse the full citation list at www .theguthealthmd.com/plantpoweredplus.

THE FOUR NUTRITION WORKHORSES

A flexible, abundant Plant Powered diet isn't just good for you—it's rigorously backed by science, powerfully anti-inflammatory, and deeply healing to your gut microbes. But can we kick it up a notch? Absolutely. There are four specific dietary components that offer supercharged healing for your microbes, gut barrier, and immune system, and they form the backbone of all Plant Powered diets. Not only do these elements stand out for their remarkable benefits but also because most of us simply aren't getting enough of them. As I've emphasized before, our goal is to boost our intake of these beneficial foods while cutting back on the harmful ones. In this chapter, we'll dive into these four power-house ingredients and explore how to integrate them into your daily routine for lasting health benefits.

Imagine for a moment that your health is a nineteenth-century wagon and these four nutrition targets are Clydesdale horses. When a person is healthy, the wagon is light and the ground is flat. It doesn't take much to get that wagon moving briskly across the plains and get someone to their destination. But when a person is dealing with a chronic inflammatory condition, now the wagon is weighed down and they're facing an uphill climb. Just one horse isn't enough to pull that heavy wagon uphill. Two are better but still not enough. If we want the strength to pull that wagon up the hill, we need the full might of all four workhorses to power the climb.

Forget dietary tribalism for a moment—our tendency to get dogmatic about certain diets. Forget the labels we apply to dietary patterns. What if I told you that the four horses are more important to your health than your dietary tribe or label? There's far more meaning in what you eat, not what you call it. Rigid dietary identities can trap us in an ideology rather than allowing us to listen to our bodies and adapt to what actually works. The goal isn't to fit into a predefined category— it's to nourish yourself in a way that supports your gut, your metabolism, and your long-term health.

Your gut microbiome is the engine that drives your health. By intentionally supplying the four key nutritional elements your body craves, you're providing premium fuel to that engine, enhancing its performance and efficiency. Importantly, there's no one-size-fits-all approach. These four nutritional categories are broad, offering flexibility and options to help you discover what works best for your unique needs. The most effective strategy is the one you'll actually stick with— tailored to your lifestyle and preferences—rather than an idealized plan that sounds perfect in theory but isn't sustainable in practice.

Let's get back to a fundamental approach. We can identify the key science-backed elements of a disease-protecting diet, but we can also create a nutrition plan that works best for us. We can eliminate the barriers and rigidity of restrictive diets to create something stronger and better. Bottom line: Own it, and make it your own. Find what works for you, but get the job done. Let's meet the four nutrition workhorses.

One: Fiber

Fiber becomes short-chain fatty acids (SCFAs). Is there a transformation more glorious? We can debate.

Grandma always said to eat more fruits and vegetables. Maybe, just maybe, Grandma was a genius.

The truth is that this shouldn't be news to you. Fruits and vegetables have a long track record of improving human health. Sure, there may be fringe parts of the internet led by quacks who ignore thousands of studies and instead make up stories about anti-nutrients and plant toxins to try to scare you into eating less of something that you're already probably not eating enough of. But if we unplug for a moment and truly listen, we'll hear the drumbeat of fruits and veggies orchestrating a quiet, confident renaissance in farmers' markets, urban gardens, community farms, and even scientific journals.

There's been a groundswell of new science building since 2006 that's fresh and exciting. It's not a change in whether or not fruits and veggies are good for you: Nearly all legitimate sources and dietary guidelines continue to recommend more fruits and veggies. What's changed is why. What once was ho-hum has taken on an aura of magic.

It's a story that I shared in my first book, *Fiber Fueled*. Plants are special foods because they have a monopoly on the healthiest nutrients— fiber, resistant starches, polyphenols, and other phytochemicals. Perhaps you've heard, I'm obsessed with fiber. I sincerely believe that it's our most pressing, most profound nutritional deficiency. Around 95 percent of America is strikingly fiber deficient. Not like marginally deficient, but majorly deficient. The average woman should consume 25 grams of fiber per day, and she gets 15. The average American man should consume 38 grams of fiber per day, and he gets 18. To meet the recommended amount, most of America needs to double its fiber intake.

But what is fiber exactly? It's not just the orange drink that Grandma had so that she could poop. I mean, it is. But it's so much more. Fiber is a carbohydrate created by nature by fusing together sugar molecules to create something much more complex. That complexity is reflected in the widely varied forms of fiber—we don't even have an estimate of how many there are. There may be millions, billions, perhaps even trillions of forms of fiber. You've likely heard fiber described as one of two types—soluble or insoluble. Soluble fiber dissolves in water to form a gel-like substance that slows digestion and also feeds gut microbes, while insoluble fiber does not dissolve and adds bulk to stool, sweeping through the colon and promoting regularity. But describing fiber as soluble or insoluble is really just our way of simplifying a topic so complex that it overwhelms even the best biochemist.

Fiber is abundant in plant-based foods—fruits, vegetables, whole grains, seeds, nuts, legumes, herbs, spices, and even mushrooms. All plants have fiber. While mushrooms are technically fungi, I like to think of them as honorary plants because of their fiber content. One place you won't find any fiber is in animal products—there's zero fiber there, a fact that's simple yet crucial to remember. Another is oil, which is 100 percent fat and therefore doesn't have any fiber.

Every plant contains various forms of fiber, including soluble and insoluble fiber. People will often ask me, "Dr. B, what's a good food to get soluble fiber?" The answer: Plants. Any of them. All of them. Don't worry about targeting specific forms of fiber. Just eat plants. They'll have what you're looking for.

So what happens when we eat plants? While most nutrients are digested and absorbed, fiber embarks on a unique journey. Humans lack the enzymes to break down fiber, allowing it to travel intact through fifteen feet of small intestine until it reaches the colon, home to thirty-eight trillion microbes. These invisible partners eagerly take over, using tens of thousands of specialized enzymes we don't possess to break down the fiber. This symbiotic relationship not only benefits the microbes but also reinforces our mutual dependence: Through our diet we provide them with fuel, and in return, they help keep us healthy.

Not all microbes wield the same enzymes: Each one plays a unique part, like musicians in a symphony, stepping up at just the right moment to perform their piece. The result of their coordinated efforts is nothing short of magical: Fiber, once indigestible, undergoes a profound metamorphosis under their skillful guidance. It emerges not as the crude fiber we started with but as beautiful, impactful short-chain fatty acids: the harmonious outcome of sweet fiber music orchestrated by our gut microbiome.

In Chapter 1, we explored the anti-inflammatory superpowers of short-chain fatty acids (SCFAs). Here's a quick summary of what we've learned so far: SCFAs empower beneficial gut microbes, prompting them to produce even more SCFAs, while suppressing harmful, inflammatory ones—tilting the balance toward healing. They activate proteins that seal and regenerate the gut barrier every three to five days and thicken the protective mucus layer lining it. By engaging special SCFA receptors, these molecules fine-tune immune cells throughout the body—whether in the bone marrow, thymus, lymph nodes, or gut lining—ensuring that both the innate and adaptive immune systems remain organized, precise, and potent. In short, SCFAs represent a principal pathway to simultaneously enhance the health of our microbes, gut barrier, and immune system. But there's more . . . Now, let's broaden our understanding of SCFAs to truly grasp just how invaluable they are.

The benefits of SCFAs extend far beyond the gut and immune systems. They trigger the release of key gut hormones like GLP-1, GIP, and peptide YY, which help regulate appetite and satiety—mechanisms that new weight-loss drugs take advantage of. They also influence hormones such as leptin, cholecystokinin, and ghrelin, which further signal fullness or hunger to the brain. Now you see why fiber and SCFAs from fiber-rich diets make you feel full and help with weight loss.

Moreover, SCFAs play a crucial role in controlling blood sugar and improving insulin sensitivity, key factors in reversing type 2 diabetes. One major mechanism is their stimulation of GLP-1 release, which prompts insulin secretion—a process mirrored by the GLP-1 drug semaglutide, used for both weight loss (Wegovy) and diabetes management (Ozempic). In addition, peptide YY and leptin assist in moving sugar from the blood into muscle and fat cells, while SCFAs activate special channels that absorb sugar into muscle and liver tissue. The net result of these coordinated actions is improved blood sugar control, which helps to maintain a healthy gut barrier, as discussed in Chapter 3.

SCFAs reduce total and LDL cholesterol and triglyceride levels by reducing cholesterol production, breaking down fatty acids, inhibiting new fat creation, and minimizing fat storage. In effect, they shift the body from fat-storage to fat-burning mode. They also keep post-meal triglycerides in check—a crucial discovery, since high triglycerides after eating are linked to cardiovascular disease and inflammation. I'll explore this further in Chapter 6 when we discuss time-restricted eating. But the point for you to lock in right now is that lower blood sugar and blood fat after meals is anti-inflammatory, and SCFAs do that for us. Additionally, SCFAs relax blood vessels and stimulate the parasympathetic nervous system, contributing to lower blood pressure. I'll delve into the benefits of parasympathetic stimulation in Chapter 8, but for now, note that SCFAs are a natural way to achieve it. All of these actions underscore why SCFAs play a pivotal role in defending against cardiovascular disease.

Consider for a moment the litany of benefits we gain from SCFAs—enhanced gut and immune function, improved blood sugar and fat control, reduced inflammation, a shift from fat storing to fat burning, and the release of satiety hormones like GLP-1. These powerful effects reveal the mechanisms that explain many of fiber's health benefits. Now let me share the health impacts highlighted in my favorite fiber study of all time.

Dr. Andrew Reynolds and his team at the University of Otago sifted through over 185 studies, tracking more than 134 million person-years of data, to see how fiber shapes our health. They found that people who ate the most fiber enjoyed markedly lower risks of dying from cardiovascular disease, coronary disease, and cancer. They were less likely to have a heart attack, stroke, or be diagnosed with diabetes or several forms of cancer—esophageal, colon, and breast. In fifty-eight clinical trials, more fiber intake produced meaningful improvements in weight loss, fat loss, total and LDL cholesterol and triglyceride levels, and blood pressure. These benefits weren't flukes or just signs of a generally healthy lifestyle—they showed a clear dose–response relationship, meaning the more fiber you eat, the greater the benefits. No surprise, when people ate more fiber, they lived longer. This compelling evidence cements fiber's role as a powerhouse nutrient, directly contributing to a longer, healthier life.

Resistant starches are essentially the same as fiber and worthy of all of the accolades that fiber gets. Their structure is different—they are starch like you find in potatoes, bananas, beans, and whole grains. But they are the same in function. Like fiber, resistant starches escape digestion in the small intestine. Like fiber, they are food for the microbiome. Like fiber, they are magically transformed into short-chain fatty acids.

All fermentable fiber and resistant starches can be broken down into a blend of acetate, propionate, and butyrate. These three SCFAs aren't totally interchangeable—certain ones do certain things. But you don't need to worry about that, as long as you follow my one simple rule. Dare I call it the Golden Rule:

EAT A VARIETY OF PLANTS.

Variety is nature's way of achieving equilibrium—it's like diversifying your stock portfolio. Different plants contain varied forms of fiber that naturally even out the balance among acetate, propionate, and butyrate. Variety naturally calibrates and optimizes the blend of SCFAs, nurturing a more resilient gut ecosystem and robust health.

But eating for variety is more than just obtaining different forms of fiber to balance SCFAs. Plants provide much more than fiber, and different plants will provide different polyphenols or healthy fats or other phytochemicals. The result is that in the American Gut Project, they found that those with the healthiest guts were the ones who ate thirty or more different plant foods per week. In *Fiber Fueled*, I called this the Golden Rule of Gut Health. It still is, and adding a wider variety of plants to your diet should be a top priority.

In this section, I'm heralding the benefits of fiber, and here's how I want you to do it. Stop counting grams of fiber. Start counting plants. Make it your goal to build toward thirty or more plants per week, and when you accomplish it, then set your goal even higher. If you eat enough different plants, you will get plenty of fiber. And you'll get various types of fiber to produce a blend of acetate, propionate, and butyrate. But you'll also get a wider variety of polyphenols. And in the next section, I'm going to show you the health benefits that come when you do that.

A Plant Powered Paradox

Y'all know I love a good paradox. Especially a good (*smirks*) plant paradox. There's something that scientists call the butyrate paradox. I've explained that butyrate promotes the creation of healthy new cells. Yet, study after study after study shows us that fiber and specifically butyrate protect us from colorectal cancer. The butyrate paradox lies in its dual role—while it promotes healthy cell renewal, it simultaneously triggers the death of cancerous cells, making it both a growth supporter and a growth fighter. How does it do both? The reason for this paradox is called the Warburg effect. Healthy cells use butyrate as their principal source of energy, rapidly eating up all the butyrate until there's little left. Cancer cells, however, use glucose (sugar) as their source of energy. Yes, sugar does in fact feed cancer. Big mistake by those indulgent cancer cells! Since they prioritize sugar over butyrate, there's extra butyrate left over to block cellular turnover and effectively kill cancer. Take that, cancer!

Myth Busters Part 1: Are Beans and Whole Grains Inflammatory Foods?

For the last twenty years, we've been given reason after reason to avoid beans and whole grains: They're not ancestral; they have anti-nutrients like phytates; lectins are the cause of our health issues; gluten causes leaky gut. The result? We've been avoiding them. The average American eats just two ounces of beans per week while consuming nine times that amount in added sugar. And while 95 percent of Americans are deficient in fiber, 98 percent of Americans are deficient in whole grains. But is our avoidance justified? Or are we being fed misinformation that's actually harming us in our food choices? My vote is for the latter. Here's why . . .

First, beans and whole grains are jam-packed with prebiotic goodness. They're about as high in fiber as you'll find. They also deliver resistant starch. And they can be a source of a third type of prebiotics, which we are about to discuss, called polyphenols. These prebiotics work together in a synergistic fashion to support the microbiome and shift it back to health.

Second, the proof is in the research. We can keep this super simple—it doesn't need to be complicated. Do beans cause inflammation? Quite the opposite. In mice with colitis, white and dark kidney beans improve gut barrier function and significantly lower inflammation. Multiple randomized controlled trials (RCTs) show that beans reduce inflammation in humans. How about whole grains? More of the same. We have literally a dozen RCTs showing less inflammation when you consume more whole grains.

Simply put, these are *not* inflammatory foods. That said, it's possible that our modern agricultural practices may explain the reports out there of people developing inflammatory health issues. Both beans and whole grains are often sprayed with glyphosate after harvest because something you use to kill weeds can also be used to kill and dry out beans and whole grains. This is why I personally opt for organic. I prefer my plants glyphosate-free. I prefer to not ingest weed killer.

Some individuals have celiac disease—an autoimmune condition where gluten triggers an immune response. If you experience symptoms when consuming gluten-containing grains, it's important to get tested. Common tests include a blood test for tissue transglutaminase (tTG) IgA antibodies, an intestinal biopsy via endoscopy, and genetic testing for HLA-DQ2 and HLA-DQ8. Additional assessments, like IgG and IgA anti-gliadin antibody tests, can indicate gluten sensitivity. If any of these tests are positive, adopting a gluten-free diet makes sense. Even if tests are negative but symptoms persist—especially if you have an autoimmune or chronic inflammatory condition—it may be worth trying a gluten-free diet to see if you feel better. However, a gluten-free diet isn't universally necessary or beneficial. In fact, research suggests that eliminating gluten-containing whole grains can increase the risk of heart disease and diabetes, so it's crucial to weigh the benefits and drawbacks before making broad dietary changes.

To summarize my thoughts on the complex topic of gluten: First, if you are experiencing symptoms related to gluten, you should be tested for celiac disease. If your test is negative, know the evidence that gluten alone triggers the immune system in non-celiac individuals is weak—mostly supported by lab studies without solid human evidence. It's possible that glyphosate, commonly sprayed on conventional wheat, could be the real culprit. This would explain why people enjoy gluten-rich foods in places like Italy without issues—another reason to choose organic. Additionally, non-gluten components of wheat, barley, and rye called fructans are known to cause digestive symptoms. This could be why many people feel better when eating sourdough bread, which naturally reduces fructan content. If you decide to go gluten-free, focus on incorporating gluten-free whole grains—such as quinoa, sorghum, teff, amaranth, buckwheat, and rice—to ensure you have a nutritious and balanced diet.

At their core, beans and whole grains are microbiome foods. More than most other plant-based foods, they powerfully feed and fuel your microbiome with fiber, resistant starch, and polyphenols. What that also means is that if you have a damaged gut, you are highly likely to struggle to digest them because these nutrients require your gut microbes in order to be digested. The result is that you might experience bloating, gas, and generally feel unwell. But bloating is not inflammation. It's sloppy digestion. Your gut is struggling to keep up with the volume of prebiotics. The solution to this is to ease into these foods. Start low, and go slow.

Sources of Fiber (Grams of Fiber per 100 Grams)

Fruits		
	Avocado	6.7
	Raspberries	6.5
	Blackberries	5.3
	Pear, with skin	3.1
	Apple, with skin	2.4

Vegetables	Artichoke, cooked	8.6
	Collard greens, cooked	4.0
	Brussels sprouts	3.8
	Sweet potato, with skin, baked	3.3
	Broccoli	2.6
Whole Grains	Oats, rolled, dry	10.1
	Whole-wheat bread	7.0
	Barley, pearled, cooked	3.8
	Quinoa, cooked	2.8
	Brown rice, cooked	1.8
Seeds and Nuts	Basil seeds	38.0
	Chia seeds	34.0
	Flaxseeds	27.0
	Almonds	12.5
	Pistachios	10.6
Legumes (cooked)	Black beans	8.7
	Lentils	7.9
	Chickpeas	7.6
	Kidney beans	6.4
	Green peas	5.5

Two: Polyphenols

Where the rainbow intersects with the pot of gold

Have you heard about polyphenols? Simply put, they are natural compounds found in plants responsible for the wide range of colors that we find in fruits and vegetables. If you're wondering where the rainbow in the produce section comes from, you have your answer. When we say, "Eat the rainbow," it's really just a way of encouraging you to consume different polyphenols.

The name "polyphenol" refers to their chemical structure. You'll also hear polyphenols referred to as antioxidants, but we're actually moving away from this as we learn more about polyphenols.

Admittedly, polyphenols are a bit of a nutritional mystery. There are a number of reasons for this. First, they are technically not considered nutrients, nor are they a source of energy. For this reason, there's no Recommended Daily Intake (or RDI) for us to judge whether our intake is adequate or inadequate. Vitamins, minerals, and even fiber have an RDI. Second, they are wildly diverse. There are over eight thousand varieties. The diversity makes it difficult to describe precisely what they are and what they do. It also makes it difficult to study them, as it requires isolation of individual polyphenols, which is quite tedious on multiple levels.

Yet, emerging from the darkness, there's a beacon of light: simple rules that guide our understanding of polyphenols and make me incredibly excited about their role in immunonutrition. Check this out:

1 **Polyphenols are found in plants.** Fruits and vegetables—*yes!* And also whole grains, seeds, nuts, and legumes. Mushrooms, our honorary plants, also contain polyphenols. Any and every time you add plants to your plate, you are adding polyphenols.

2 **Every plant will offer a diverse mix of polyphenols.** This polyphenol fingerprint is unique to the plant species. It may overlap in some ways with other plant foods, but it's important to recognize each plant has a unique blend of polyphenols.

3 **A total of 90 to 95 percent of polyphenols require help from your gut microbes to be absorbed.** Polyphenols are large and chemically complex, which means they can't be easily absorbed. They escape digestion and concentrate in the colon, where gut microbes snap their little wizard wands and—*boom*—make the

polyphenols bioactive and ready for absorption. Fermentation has a similar effect on polyphenols as gut microbes, transforming them to make them more bioavailable.

4 **Polyphenols support a healthy gut microbiome.** They suppress pathogens. For example, the polyphenol resveratrol suppresses *Salmonella enterica*, *Enterococcus faecalis*, and *E. coli*. They also nurture beneficial microbes. Red wine polyphenols increase *Bifidobacterium*, *Lactobacillus*, *Faecalibacterium prausnitzii*, and *Roseburia*. Notably, the same benefits were provided by alcohol-free red wine. It's the fermented polyphenols, not the alcohol. An important addition to what I said in Chapter 3: You don't need alcohol to get the benefits of red wine!

5 **We should strive toward consuming a diverse mix of poly-phenols.** Every plant contains a mix of polyphenols. Every polyphenol has unique health benefits, both for you and for your gut microbes. Because polyphenols are so numerous and so complex, it's difficult for us to study them in isolation and there's a lot that we don't know. But what we *do* know is that if you eat a wide variety of plants, you will be naturally consuming a broader variety of polyphenols to provide their healing effects: more evidence for the Golden Rule.

Okay, is it just me, or do the polyphenols sound a bit like fiber? Like fiber, they are found in plants, they have diverse chemical structures, they are not absorbed or active until they come into contact with our gut bugs, and then they impact the gut microbiome and create healing effects throughout the body.

It's true. They *do* sound an awful lot like fiber, only they're different: different chemical structure; different enzymes to activate them; different effects on the gut barrier, immune system, and body. So let's not treat them the same. But they also don't exist in a separate universe. They're right there, working alongside and in collaboration with fiber.

In fact, fiber and polyphenols are synergistic contributors to the production of our precious anti-inflammatory SCFAs. Imagine for a moment that we have a factory (our gut) that produces the world's greatest anti-inflammatory commodity—short-chain fatty acids. Fiber is our raw material. We need the fiber to manufacture the SCFAs. Without the fiber, the factory is an empty shell, sad and without purpose. A sprinkle of fiber is magic. Start adding fiber, and suddenly the lights power on, the gates of the factory open, and some of the local workers file in, eager to work. But here's where the polyphenols come in. They are the world's best HR department, offering you the ability to organize and recruit the perfect mix of workers for that factory. Now, thanks to the polyphenols, you have a factory staffed with an enthusiastic, SCFA-loving crew of gut microbes that are eager and excited to help you maximally produce your SCFAs. Focused and coordinated, the factory becomes not only a well-oiled machine that cranks out as many SCFAs as they can squeeze out of the raw ingredient (fiber), but also a happy place, filled with enthusiastic workers who love being there and love contributing to the success of the factory. By including polyphenols with your fiber, you're able to increase the efficiency of your gut factory and squeeze more SCFAs out of your fiber. Same fiber, more efficiency, more SCFAs: That's a winning combination.

Now, what *exactly* do they do to the immune system? Well, it's all a bit complex. Let's start with the foundation—more SCFAs. As we know, SCFAs are our anti-inflammatory superheroes because they impact the microbes, the barrier, and the immune system. So, thank you, polyphenols, for providing more superhero SCFAs.

Polyphenols may also have individual properties or effects in the body, including on the immune system or on different organs in the body. Characterizing these individual properties is a great challenge, as you can't paint with broad strokes when there are thousands of polyphenols and what we're describing is specific to individual or classes of polyphenols. Also, it depends on the makeup of your gut microbiome, which is highly personalized and ever evolving. But suffice it to say that the evidence that we have to date, and what we expect to continue to emerge in the years to come, shows us that polyphenols are anti-inflammatory powerhouses.

Let me give you an example. Lingonberry, cranberries, red grapes, strawberries, and blueberries contain groups of polyphenols called proanthocyanidins. It's where their bold, powerful red, blue, and purple colors come from. Well, when our gut bacteria come into contact with proanthocyanidins, they transform them into several different new metabolites that are anti-inflammatory, reducing TNF-α, IL-1β, and IL-6 release when immune cells come into contact with LPS. Similar effects have been seen with polyphenols called hydroxycinnamic acid derivatives found in carrots, eggplant, cabbage, and artichokes, or caffeic acid derivatives found in apples, spinach, and black chokeberry.

Let's take a closer look at lingonberries. Way up north, where only the strong survive the harsh winters, you'll find small but resilient evergreen shrubs that produce red lingonberry fruit twice a year, once in the spring and once in the summer. The lingonberry tastes bitter like a cranberry and is the size of a wild blueberry. The bitterness comes from the gush of polyphenols. Lingonberries don't just survive in this harsh environment; they thrive. In fact, the stress they grow under actually activates survival mechanisms that instigate copious production of polyphenols. Pressure molds the diamond, and what results is a thing of beauty. Environmentally challenged lingonberries have the highest polyphenol content among all berries. What this has taught us is that harsh conditions power the production of polyphenols. Plants that grow under stressful conditions, like wild and organic plants, have more polyphenols than greenhouse-cultivated ones do. As Dr. Sharon Bergquist explains in *The Stress Paradox*, a life utterly free of challenges isn't necessarily better—in nature, as in our lives, stress can be the very spark that ignites resilience and growth.

Scientists have wondered about the effects of polyphenols on the immune system, so, naturally, they studied the lingonberry. Twelve polyphenols from lingonberry were tested with macrophages. Macrophages are an immune cell that, depending on the environment, can produce inflammation or suppress it. At a branch point where the macrophages could go either way—pro- or anti-inflammatory—the lingonberry polyphenols were pushing the macrophages to be anti-inflammatory.

What happens when you eat a whole bunch of high-polyphenol plants? In the MAPLE trial they took a group of elderly adults with a broken gut barrier and randomized them to either a high polyphenol diet or a control diet. What they found was that over the course of eight weeks, those eating the high polyphenol diet experienced a significant improvement in their gut barrier function. By the way, as proof of what I've been saying, they also found that the high polyphenol diet increased the prevalence of the butyrate-producing bacteria. It's all starting to come together now!

The takeaway is that different plants have different polyphenols, and more stressed-out plants will have more polyphenols. Thanks to our gut bugs, these polyphenols impact our immune cells and tone down inflammation. When we eat a wide variety of plants in many different colors, we expose our microbiome to many kinds of both polyphenols and fiber and get the most out of the synergistic benefits that they provide.

Myth Busters Part 2: Are Nightshades Problematic?

You've heard that nightshades are a serious problem for people who have autoimmune diseases. What's the story there? Nightshades are plants in the Solanaceae family, of which there are more than three thousand varieties. The ones you most commonly eat are tomatoes, potatoes, peppers (all varieties), and eggplant. Many believe they cause inflammation due to the presence of glycoalkaloids. Admittedly, if you purified and isolated glycoalkaloids, they would definitely be dangerous. It's believed that a nightshade herb called belladonna was the poison that Juliet used to fake her death in Shakespeare's classic play. But purified and isolated glycoalkaloids are NOT what you're eating when you enjoy tomatoes or potatoes. And glycoalkaloids are a very small part of the bigger nutritional profile of these foods that include fiber and polyphenols. So what happens when you actually eat these foods?

The aggregate result of seven clinical trials was that eating tomatoes lowers your TNF-α levels. In another study, tomatoes led to beneficial changes in the gut microbiome that lowered intestinal inflammation markers. Consumption of yellow potatoes and particularly purple potatoes reduced inflammatory cytokine levels, and this was attributed to the polyphenol content in the colored potatoes. Epidemiology studies associate hot pepper consumption with longevity and less death from heart disease.

Here's the bottom line: Avoid eating green potatoes, as they're unsafe, and don't overindulge in hot peppers to the point of causing diarrhea. But for most people, nightshade vegetables can be enjoyed without fear. If you firmly believe a particular food triggers symptoms, trust your instincts—it's perfectly reasonable to reduce or eliminate that one specific item. But let's strive not to cut out broad categories of plants. Instead, focus on expanding your fruit and vegetable variety to ensure you're getting the full spectrum of nutrients and benefits.

Sources of Polyphenols (Milligrams of Polyphenols per 100 Grams)

Red **(anthocyanins)**	Lingonberry	560
	Cranberries	525
	Cherries	274
	Raspberries	250
	Strawberries	235
Orange/Yellow **(flavones, flavonols, flavanones)**	Mango	170
	Orange	100
	Apricot	55
	Peach	50
	Pineapple	47
Green **(catechins, flavonols)**	Matcha green tea, powdered	3,000
	Green olives	330
	Green apple	136
	Spinach	119
	Green grapes	100
Blue/Purple **(anthocyanins)**	Blueberries	560
	Blackberries	260
	Plums	247
	Purple cabbage	168
	Eggplant, with skin	110

Three: Healthy Fat

Perhaps surprisingly great for the gut

For many years, we've been told that all fats are bad—they're villains lurking in our meals, ready to clog arteries and harm our health. But as we've learned through careful scientific research, the truth is more nuanced. Not all fats are created equal. Different types of fats behave differently in the body, and their impact can vary dramatically depending on their source and composition. This is particularly relevant when considering the health of our gut microbes and the delicate balance of our internal ecosystem.

Of the four main types of dietary fats—trans fats, saturated fats, monounsaturated fats (MUFAs), and polyunsaturated fats (PUFAs)—reducing trans and saturated fats is wise, especially when consumed in excess. As discussed in Chapter 3, these fats can contribute to inflammation and chronic disease when not kept in check. But MUFAs and PUFAs are a different story.

Monounsaturated Fatty Acids (MUFAs)

MUFAs are found abundantly in olives and extra-virgin olive oil (EVOO) as well as in nuts and avocados. Animal products may also contain MUFAs, but there's an important catch: Animal-based MUFAs tend to ride alongside saturated fats, which muddies the health picture. Research by Dr. Frank Hu, a renowned Harvard scientist, shows that replacing saturated fat, refined carbohydrates, and trans fats with plant-based MUFAs reduces heart disease risk by 17 percent, 14 percent, and 20 percent, respectively. This benefit did not hold true for animal-based MUFAs. In fact, if you swap out both animal-based MUFAs and saturated fats for plant-based MUFAs, you can cut heart disease risk by about 19 percent. The takeaway here is that not all MUFAs are the same: Plant-based sources are clearly preferred.

The benefits of MUFAs extend beyond heart health. In a study examining people with rheumatoid arthritis (RA), those with RA were shown to consume significantly fewer MUFAs, leaning instead on saturated fats. After controlling for other factors, researchers identified a strong trend linking higher MUFA intake to remission of RA symptoms, and subsequent work confirmed the role of MUFAs in reducing RA-related inflammation.

This aligns seamlessly with the Mediterranean diet, whose champion—extra-virgin olive oil (EVOO)—strides into the arena like a Roman gladiator, armed with polyphenols and ready to conquer inflammation. Consider the distinctive peppery, bitter taste of a high-quality EVOO—it burns! Those flavor notes come from a complex blend of polyphenols. Embrace that bitterness! It's not just a quirky flavor; these polyphenols pack a significant health boost. EVOO has consistently proven beneficial for the gut microbiome in human studies. In one trial, daily EVOO consumption over twelve weeks led to improved gut diversity among male participants and an increase in beneficial bacteria like *Akkermansia* in female participants. The polyphenols in EVOO act like powerful prebiotics, supporting a healthier gut ecosystem.

How to Select the Best EVOO

The polyphenol content of extra-virgin olive oil can vary widely, from 40 milligrams up to 530 milligrams per kilogram of oil. Clearly, we'd prefer to be on the higher end of that spectrum. To help accomplish this, there are a few tricks:

1. **Make sure it's extra-virgin olive oil.** This is the highest quality and retains the most polyphenols because it's mechanically pressed rather than refined with heat or chemicals.

2. **Look for brands that disclose polyphenol content.** Some bottles will clearly list their polyphenol levels, while others may provide lab reports upon request and often provide a QR code on the bottle.

3. **Choose cold pressed, and when possible consume it at room temperature.** High heat degrades many polyphenols.

4. **Check the expiration date.** In general, olive oil is freshest in the first nine months after pressing.

5. **Check the olives in the bottle.** Much like wine is assigned to specific grapes, so is olive oil. The olives with the highest polyphenol content are Coratina, Conicabra, Koroneiki, Moraiolo, and Picual. You can bring this book to the supermarket or add a little note to your phone for when you're in the EVOO aisle.

6. **When in doubt, buy Italian.** In a study of olive oil from nine countries, Italian EVOO consistently came out on top. Congratulazioni!

7. **Embrace the bitter taste!** The bitterness comes from the polyphenols.

8. **A dark glass bottle is preferred** to protect the oil from sun damage.

Foods High in MUFAs (Grams of MUFA per 100 Grams)

Nuts and Seeds	Macadamia nuts	58.9
	Hazelnuts	45.7
	Almonds	31.6
	Cashews	23.8
	Peanuts	24.7
Fruits and Vegetables	Black olives	11.0
	Avocado	9.8
	Green olives	8.3

Oils	Olive oil (extra-virgin)	73.0
	Olive oil (non-extra-virgin)	72.0
	Avocado oil	70.6
Animal-Based	Cheddar cheese	9.0
	Ground beef, cooked	8.6
	Pork chop, cooked	5.7
	Salmon	5.6
	Chicken thigh (with skin, cooked)	5.2

Polyunsaturated Fatty Acids (PUFAs)

Polyunsaturated fatty acids (PUFAs) are vital for controlling inflammation, and surprisingly, they all originate from plants. While fish oil and salmon are often cited as prime PUFA sources, the truth is that these benefits trace back to plant life. For example, the omega-3 fats found in fish begin their journey in sea plants like algae and plankton. As these fats move up the food chain, they concentrate in larger marine life, yet their origin remains unmistakably plant-based. PUFAs are just as Plant Powered as fiber and polyphenols, and recognizing their plant roots reinforces the idea that the healthiest nutrients—no matter how they appear to us—ultimately come from the plant world.

Among PUFAs, omega-3 fats stand out. They are our anti-inflammatory fat. There are three main types of omega-3s: ALA (alpha-linolenic acid), EPA (eicosapentaenoic acid), and DHA (docosahexaenoic acid). Much like acetate, propionate, and butyrate have a different number of carbon molecules—2, 3, and 4, respectively—so too do ALA, EPA, and DHA: 18, 20, and 22, respectively. The three are similar, but they are not the same.

EPA and even more so DHA are the most important. They carry potent anti-inflammatory powers—they calm cytokines, boost IL-10 (an anti-inflammatory signal), and work directly on immune cells to cool them off. DHA is especially important for the brain, which is about 60 percent fat by weight, with DHA as the most abundant fatty acid in there.

So how do we get them? ALA is found in seeds and nuts—chia seeds, flaxseeds, hempseeds, basil seeds, and walnuts. EPA and DHA mainly come from marine plants, fish (particularly fatty fish), shellfish, and bivalves. Our body has enzymes to convert ALA into EPA and EPA into DHA. In theory, if you simply consume lots of ALA-rich seeds and nuts, you'd be able to fulfill your EPA and DHA requirements. But in the real world, the conversion is woefully inefficient, yielding inadequate amounts of DHA (the most critical one) for most.

RATES OF CONVERSION OF ALA TO OTHER FORMS OF OMEGA-3 FATS	PREMENOPAUSAL WOMEN	YOUNG MEN
EPA	21%	9%
DHA	8%	4% or less

Estrogen likely plays a role here, which explains why premenopausal women tend to have higher DHA levels. Along with many other changes, this benefit goes away at menopause.

The anti-inflammatory benefits of omega-3s also tie directly into their effects in the gut. In a randomized, controlled diet intervention study, researchers found that as blood levels of DHA increased, leaky gut decreased. Short-chain fatty acid levels were the only thing more powerful in correcting leaky gut. Makes sense, right? Well, try this on for size: One of the ways omega-3s improve gut health is by increasing SCFA levels. Omega-3s are not precursors to SCFAs like fiber is, but much like polyphenols, they have the ability to change the gut bacteria so that you could consume the same amount of fiber and actually get even more SCFAs. What this means is that we want to pair fiber with omega-3s for the win. Even better if we can get some polyphenols in there to amplify it further.

Real-world examples bear this out. Omega-3 intake has been shown to protect against inflammatory bowel diseases like Crohn's disease and reduce the risk of developing rheumatoid arthritis. For those already living with RA, having just two servings of fish per week is associated with reduced joint inflammation. And here's an interesting one: Pregnant women who consume adequate EPA and DHA lower the risk of allergic diseases—like food allergies, asthma, rhinitis, and eczema—in their children. The authors concluded that "Omega-3 long-chain-PUFA intake during pregnancy may offer the *best opportunity* for a primary prevention strategy, decreasing the burden of allergic disease for future generations."

Yet despite these clear benefits, we're falling short on omega-3 intake. Only about 68 percent of adults meet the recommended intake, and in kids it's a mere 5 percent. Seafood—especially oily fish like salmon, herring, sardines, and cod—is the richest dietary source of EPA and DHA. Oysters are also an outstanding source, delivering not just omega-3s but also other key nutrients that can be tough to get from a vegan diet. But if you hear someone talking about omega-3s in beef, you can ignore it. Wild-caught salmon has one hundred times more omega-3 than grass-fed beef and five hundred times more omega-3 than ground beef.

Should We Be Concerned About Microplastics and Nanoplastics in Seafood?

As mentioned in Chapter 3, microplastics and nanoplastics are synthetic pollutants now found in almost every corner of our planet—accumulating in our air and our water, not just in our landfills. They've infiltrated our oceans, harming marine life and contaminating fish, shellfish, and bivalves. If our food is sick, how can it make us healthy? By ignoring how our actions disrupt nature, we now find that tiny plastic particles are detectable in human urine, stool, blood, and even organs. Though we don't yet know the full impact on our health, it's safe to say they're not doing us any favors.

While scientists work to clarify the exact risks, a cautious approach is wise. There are a few things to consider. First, nanoplastics bioaccumulate as you climb up the food chain, meaning larger fish can have higher concentrations. This is an argument to eat lower on the food chain. Second, pollution levels vary by location, making cleaner water (like remote parts of the ocean or pristine mountain streams) preferable. A healthy ecosystem creates healthy food. Third, microplastics aren't limited to seafood: Land animals and even plant-based foods can be affected, especially when processed. The honest truth is that we can't perfectly predict which foods are most contaminated. We don't even have reliable test methods. That said, this is why we begin with plant-based protein as our foundation. If you do include seafood, choose it thoughtfully, opting for cleaner waters, lower in the food chain, and more responsible sourcing whenever possible.

Foods High in Omega-3s (Grams of Omega-3 per 100 Grams)

Plant-Based (Terrestrial)— ALA Only	Flaxseeds	22.8
	Chia seeds	17.8
	Walnuts	9.1
	Hempseeds	8.7
	Basil seeds	6.5
Plant-Based (Sea)— ALA and EPA	Spirulina	0.8
	Chlorella	0.4
	Nori	0.3
	Wakame	0.2
	Dulse	0.2

Fish— EPA and DHA	Atlantic mackerel	2.6
	Atlantic salmon	2.3
	Pacific herring	2.0
	Anchovies	1.8
	Sardines	1.5
Shellfish— EPA and DHA	Oysters	1.2
	Mussels	1.0
	Scallops	0.3
	Shrimp	0.3
	Clams	0.2
Animal-Based (Terrestrial)— Mix of ALA, EPA, and DHA	Flax-fed omega-3 enriched egg	0.26
	Grass-fed beef	0.15
	Grain-fed beef	0.1
	Conventional egg	0.07
	Chicken	0.05

Of course, not everyone feels comfortable eating seafood. Allergies, personal ethics, and environmental concerns are all valid reasons to avoid or moderate it. Fortunately, you have options that allow you to align your health with your values. If you choose a vegetarian or vegan path, focus on increasing ALA intake by regularly consuming chia seeds, flaxseeds, hempseeds, basil seeds, and walnuts. Blending these into a daily omega-3 smoothie is one tasty way to do this. You can also improve the conversion of ALA to EPA and DHA by limiting omega-6 fats, which compete with omega-3s for conversion. This means avoiding oils like safflower, sunflower, corn, soybean, and grapeseed. Consider algae-based DHA/EPA supplements as well. They are a little more expensive than fish oil but are also easier in terms of maintaining purity. Some ethically minded people choose to consume bivalves—oysters, mussels, clams, and scallops—to help keep their DHA and EPA levels up. But ultimately, knowledge is power, which is why I believe in omega-3 testing. If your blood test shows adequate levels of

DHA and EPA, then you are good to go. And if these fats are deficient, then you should consider dietary changes and supplements. More on that in Chapter 7.

Whether you choose carefully sourced seafood or an algae-based supplement, or you are thoughtfully incorporating bivalves or ALA-rich seeds into your routine, the science is clear: Omega-3s matter. They matter for your gut, your heart, your brain, and your long-term health.

Myth Busters Part 3: There's More to the Story with Seed Oils and Omega-6 PUFAs

Omega-6s are the "other" PUFAs. In Chapter 3, I mentioned that they are found concentrated in our ultra-processed foods due to the liberal use of seed oils for cheap calories and flavor. There are dietary camps that would lead you to believe that the main nutritional problem that we have in the United States is our consumption of seed oils. The concern is that while omega-3s are anti-inflammatory, omega-6s may be pro-inflammatory. However, in Chapter 3, I shared the unbiased evidence that saturated fats are more inflammatory than omega-6 PUFAs and that inflammation from seed oils is typically the result of overconsumption and weight gain, which they are particularly prone to cause when bundled with UPFs that are hyperpalatable.

Does this mean seed oils are off the hook and falsely attacked? Not exactly. The problem that we have, much like our consumption of saturated fat, is the absence of balance in our diet. Our diet is deficient in omega-3s and simultaneously oversaturated with seed oils, resulting in the average American consuming fifteen to twenty times more omega-6s than they do omega-3s. This number would be four to one or less if we consumed an unprocessed diet because ratios of fifteen to one or worse do not exist in nature and exist only when engineered by humans.

One additional significant source of omega-6 fatty acids warrants acknowledgment: arachidonic acid. This particular fat is predominantly found in meat and eggs and is generally absent from plant-based foods. In a study involving people with rheumatoid arthritis, participants who minimized their intake of arachidonic acid—primarily by reducing meat consumption and supplementing with fish oil—experienced fewer tender and swollen joints. Balance is key and can be attained by simply eating more plants—containing fiber and polyphenols—and emphasizing omega-3s.

I have to make one thing perfectly clear: I'm not a fan of seed oils. There are many issues. They oxidize at high heat, producing toxic chemicals. Cooking french fries in seed oils is a terrible mistake, although switching to beef tallow isn't any better. The industrial production of seed oils often involves high heat, chemical solvents, and deodorization, which leave behind harmful chemicals and less beneficial compounds. Lastly, seed oils may concentrate contaminants like pesticide residues and heavy metals.

So while I don't think seed oils are the principal cause of our problems, I do have a problem with seed oils. My preference is EVOO at cooler temperatures and rare use of avocado oil at higher temperatures.

Four: Fermented Foods

Our little microbial wizards cast a spell that transforms the power of our food.

Long before humans existed, microbes were little wizards, whipping their wands and transforming their environment. This includes playing a central role in the life cycle of our food, from soil to seed to fruit to decomposition and back to soil. Within that cycle is the opportunity for fermentation, a process where bacteria and yeasts convert sugar into energy for themselves and, in doing so, transform the food while producing other bioactive chemicals. Our prehistoric ancestors surely stumbled upon slightly fizzy overripe fruit, alcohol from fermented honey, curds from milk. Spontaneous fermentation is a part of nature, whether humans are present or not.

But across the globe—on every continent—all cultures eventually discovered techniques that, when applied to natural food sources in their ecosystem, would result in preservation and enhanced food safety, not to mention more complex flavors. Cabbage became bubbling pots of spicy kimchi in Korea and tangy sauerkraut in Eastern Europe; wild yeast and grains along the Nile became sourdough bread in ancient Egypt; and goat and sheep farmers in the Caucasus Mountains of Eurasia stumbled upon tangy milk, which we now call kefir. Fermentation reflects the ingenuity of cultures adapting to their landscapes. Little did they realize that there were these magical little bugs, too small to see, that were powering these transformations. Can you imagine how crazy that would seem to them?

Fermentation proved indispensable as tribal settlements grew into flourishing civilizations. By extending the life of perishable foods, we could transition from nomadic hunters and gatherers to settled agricultural communities. This is foundational to human civilization. By naturally suppressing pathogens in food, we enhanced food safety and protected ourselves from life-threatening infections. Of course, the exciting new flavors that we unlocked—tangy, effervescent, complex, and sometimes funky—became naturally woven into our collective culinary heritage and celebrated for generations to come. As we spread, settled, and built societies across continents, these practices evolved and diversified. Each culture, in its own unique way, integrated fermentation into its traditions—so much so that, over millennia, we effectively shaped our evolution alongside these microbial allies.

Common Ferments and Their Area of Origin

Sauerkraut (China/Eastern Europe)

Kimchi (Korea)

Pickles (Eastern Europe)

Miso (Japan)

Tempeh (Indonesia)

Kombucha (China)

Sourdough bread (Ancient Egypt)

Yogurt (Middle East)

Various cheeses (Worldwide)

Kefir (Caucasus region)

Beer (Ancient Mesopotamia)

Wine (Caucasus Region/ Georgia)

Olives (Mediterranean)

Natto (Japan)

Fish sauce (Southeast Asia)

Chocolate (Mesoamerica)

Fermentation is a magical transformation driven by microbes using enzymes like spells. As microbes work, they consume simple sugars and produce organic acids that lower the pH, creating an environment inhospitable to spoilage organisms. At the same time, some sugars are reassembled into special prebiotic fibers known as exopolysaccharides, resulting in less sugar and more beneficial compounds. Moreover, these microbes convert starch into resistant starch, the starch equivalent of prebiotic fiber. In essence, fermentation overhauls carbohydrates by reducing their sugar content and boosting their prebiotic value.

It's not just carbohydrates undergoing transformation. Microbes also have digestive enzymes that break down protein into smaller pieces and anti-nutrients get removed, making protein absorption easier. Some of the protein becomes bioactive peptides, such as fermented dairy that contains ACE inhibitor peptides that naturally lower blood pressure. Fats get changed, too. Microbes have enzymes capable of reducing and transforming fats, converting them into healthier forms. For example, during fermentation, full-fat dairy undergoes a reduction in saturated fat and an increase in conjugated linoleic acid (CLA), a healthy fat that is anti-inflammatory.

All three macronutrients—carbs, proteins, and fats—change and get better through fermentation. Microbial enzymes also unlock polyphenols, making them more available and enhancing their potential impact once consumed. Similarly, B vitamins, including the elusive vitamin B_{12}, are produced. Minerals like zinc, iron, and calcium become more readily absorbed because anti-nutrients like phytates get reduced. Gluten, FODMAPs (fermentable oligosaccharides, disaccharides, monosaccharides, and polyols), and even pesticide residues are reduced as well. Collectively, these transformations provide a glimpse into a microscopic world where tiny, unseen wizards put their wands to work to enhance the properties of our food.

Who Needs to Be Cautious When Eating Fermented Foods?

There's no one-size-fits-all in nutrition. You have to match your choices to your personal needs. With that in mind, people who have histamine intolerance or a history of migraines may need to reduce or temporarily eliminate fermented foods because they are naturally high in histamine and other biogenic amines. In those with histamine intolerance, fermented foods might trigger bloating, nasal congestion, headaches, brain fog, skin rashes, or other symptoms. I discussed histamine intolerance and have a protocol for it in *The Fiber Fueled Cookbook*, so if you deal with this health issue, then check that book out. The key with histamine intolerance is to heal the gut barrier, which is what we're doing in this book.

Additionally, many fermented vegetables are high in salt. Although the limited evidence does not indicate worsening of blood pressure, it's prudent for those with high blood pressure or chronic kidney disease to be cautious.

There are several important and fascinating properties of fermented foods:

First, a ferment is an ecosystem of its own, much like our gut. A delicious ferment is the product of a healthy ecosystem that's thriving and in balance. So *of course* it would be good for us to absorb this healthy ecosystem into our own. You've heard me say: "If our food is sick, how can it make us healthy?" Now we're revisiting that, from the other side, where we see an opportunity to invite a healthy ecosystem to merge with our own.

Second, fermentation is a form of predigestion. What's happening outside the body mirrors what happens inside the body. The difference is that the outside microbes are given extra time, which allows them to tactically transform our food in ways that makes life extremely easy for our inside microbes.

Third, fermentation is also a form of slow cooking, which in my opinion always produces the most delicious food. "Cooking" is defined as the process of deliberately modifying raw ingredients into prepared foods, which is what we're doing here. These microbes are wearing two hats—a wizard hat *and* a chef's hat.

Fourth, fermentation is a powerful tool for gut health created by Mother Nature. It boosts exopolysaccharides and resistant starch. Polyphenols become more bioavailable. It lowers sugar and pesticide residues. Fats and proteins are transformed into anti-inflammatory goodness. Mother Nature is giving us *exactly* what we need. Nature has more intelligence than we do, and this is an opportunity for us to both celebrate and take advantage of that.

What do we know about the impact of fermented foods on your gut microbes and immune system? In an analysis of nearly seven thousand people, one study found that those who regularly consumed fermented foods had microbes from their ferments showing up in their microbiome analysis. In a separate study, some of my friends at Stanford University—Professors Christopher Gardner, Erica Sonnenburg, and

Justin Sonnenburg—asked people to ramp up their fermented food intake. Eight weeks later, their gut microbiome had significantly more diversity than when they started. A more diverse microbiome is a more stable, resilient microbiome. The increase in gut diversity didn't just suddenly pop up at eight weeks; with every two-week measurement, it ramped up. As gut diversity went up, inflammation went down. There were nineteen different measures of inflammation that declined with regular consumption of fermented foods. What this means is that if we make the choice to add more fermented foods to our plates, we can expect that consistency will be rewarded. For the participants in the study, from Day 1 up to Day 56 (eight weeks), each day their gut got a little stronger, which translates into a stronger gut barrier, allowing the immune system the space it needs to settle down, and their body became less inflamed. By nurturing their gut with fermented foods, they were actively turning down the dial on chronic inflammation—something we all have the power to do. As we talk more about how to heal the gut and your immune system, we will return to the findings from this study in Chapter 9. Lock this one in your brain now.

Myth Busters Part 4: Is Dairy Inflammatory?

We've all heard that dairy products are inflammatory, and yet fermented dairy such as yogurt or kefir appears in many healthy dietary patterns from across the globe. What is the real story about dairy and how does fermented dairy change the picture?

In a systematic review of fifty-two randomized controlled trials, fermented dairy was found to have an anti-inflammatory effect. In a four-week study of inflammatory bowel disease, drinking kefir twice a day was associated with beneficial changes in the gut microbiome, lower inflammatory measures, and fewer gut symptoms in those with Crohn's disease. And in the eight-week aforementioned fermented food study from Stanford University, the number one food for increasing gut diversity was yogurt.

But just as seed oils may reduce inflammation compared to saturated fats, yet come with concerns about oxidation and processing, I have similar reservations about dairy products—including fermented ones. First, many dairy cows are treated with recombinant bovine growth hormone (rBGH) or recombinant bovine somatotropin (rBST) to boost milk production, which has been linked to hormonal imbalances and potential cancer risks (though research is mixed). Even in cows not treated with artificial hormones, naturally occurring hormones in milk can still influence our bodies. For example, estrogens in milk have been shown to lower testosterone levels in men and children. Similarly, dairy intake may impact women's estrogen levels and potentially their fertility. Additionally, dairy cows are routinely given antibiotics to prevent infections like mastitis, which contributes to antibiotic resistance, and residues can be detected in milk. Buying organic dairy reduces exposure to antibiotics and artificial hormones, but naturally occurring hormones remain.

There are ethical concerns surrounding dairy production, and I leave those for each of us to consider. From a health standpoint, if dairy is part of your diet, fermented dairy is the most beneficial choice. By no means am I suggesting that you increase your dairy intake or reintroduce it if you've already removed it. There are some people who believe that dairy products make their inflammatory or autoimmune disease worse, and if so, it should be avoided. That said, if you do choose to consume dairy, fermented options—preferably those with live active cultures—offer the greatest potential health benefits due to their probiotics and improved digestibility.

Focus on the Four Horses

Stop worrying about restrictive lists and tribalistic diets with rigid rules, and instead concentrate on a Plant Powered diet built on the four workhorses: fiber, polyphenols, healthy fats, and fermented foods. These are our nonnegotiables. We *need* to have them. Every meal is an opportunity to include these on your plate and let them do the work for you. These four categories offer a profoundly simple and effective approach that acknowledges our evolved connections between diet, gut, and immunity and sets the stage for true healing. It's so basic: Get back to wholesome, minimally processed foods and get out of the way because the body wants to heal.

Chapter 5 is backed by 206 references gathered through an extensive review of the scientific literature. You can browse the full citation list at www .theguthealthmd.com/plantpoweredplus.

TIMING IS EVERYTHING

Leveraging Our Circadian Rhythm

I talk a lot about the power of nutrition for healing the gut with my patients and anyone else who will listen. But our microbes actually have a lot of different needs, not just what we feed them. I remember talking with Melinda, a thirty-three-year-old woman who had been battling ulcerative colitis for several years. She would show up to my clinic slumped over, head in her hands, barely able to keep her eyes open. Despite trying various treatments for her condition, we were struggling to get it under control. When it flared up, she had urgent, sometimes bloody diarrhea, day and night, plus cramping and abdominal pain that would build until there was an explosion. I knew diet was something we needed to consider, as well as medication, but I also knew she worked as a line cook at a busy restaurant downtown, so most nights she was going hard until midnight. When I suggested we work together to get her circadian rhythm back on track, she was surprised. "You think my crazy schedule is making my colitis worse?"

"It *definitely* is a factor. Is it the only thing? No. But when we get you back in rhythm, get your daily schedule realigned with how your body is meant to work, I think you're going to notice a difference. You will literally feel it. The results will speak for themselves."

Restoring Melinda's internal clock centered on three key lifestyle adjustments that tap into her natural biorhythms and synchronize them with her daily routine to optimize both her and her microbes. These three main strategies to restore her circadian rhythm worked for her, and they can work for you:

1. More light in the morning, less light in the evening.

2. Tight mealtimes, only during daylight.

3. Sleep consistency.

As you move through this chapter, I want you to keep in mind one word, the key word for circadian rhythm—CONSISTENCY. This is what it ultimately boils down to.

The Body's Daily Symphony to Harmonize Your Health

Our circadian rhythm is our daily biological clock. It is the way in which our body keeps time and tries to best serve our needs. You see, your body performs its different functions like sleeping, eating, digesting, and physical activity best when it can synchronize them in a consistent, rhythmic pattern. Imagine that your body is like an orchestra and your organs are like different musical instruments. When we synchronize them, the result is beautiful, harmonious music. But step into the middle school band practice and what you hear may be something quite different. Their rhythmic disarray is chaotic, disjointed, and frankly cringeworthy. Synchronization is necessary to make sweet, sweet music. After all, it isn't the instruments that make the difference but the synchronization—why we happily pay top dollar for a world-class symphony yet wince through the same instruments in a disjointed school band. Timing is everything.

When our circadian rhythm is aligned, our body has a schedule for the day. It understands what we plan to do and when we plan to do it, and it can synchronize our organs and their functions so that they're all working together, in harmony, to fulfill that daily schedule like sweet, sweet music.

The conductor of our bodily orchestra is called the suprachiasmatic nucleus, or SCN. The SCN is a cluster of nerves in our brain that is perfectly positioned to collect information from both eyes. The SCN wants to understand where we are in our twenty-four-hour clock so it can optimally coordinate our bodily functions. The way it does this is by measuring the amount of light that hits our eyes' retinas. There's a certain time when light starts and when light ends, and that allows the body to distinguish between day and night. Your body evolved an internal clock that resets every twenty-four hours, corresponding to the rise and fall of the sun. The SCN uses two main hormones—cortisol and melatonin—to coordinate with the rest of the body. These hormones are a bit like yin and yang. Cortisol is your get-up-and-go hormone. Melatonin is your slow-down-and-sleep hormone. By controlling these hormones, the SCN is able to better orchestrate our circadian rhythm in the same way that a driver controls a car with a gas pedal and a brake—or, to keep with my original metaphor, in the same way a conductor is able to drive the tempo into a lively, fast allegro or ease into a slow adagio. NASCAR meets Beethoven—I didn't see that one coming.

The balance of these hormones influences much more than whether we are sleepy or alert. While you are awake, cortisol helps support and coordinate functions like eating, digestion, movement, focus, performing cognitive tasks, socializing, and pooping. Melatonin doesn't just help you fall asleep; it also helps your brain consolidate memories, your metabolism recalibrate, and your body heal. Yin and yang: When melatonin levels go up, cortisol levels go down; cortisol is at its highest between 7:00 and 8:00 a.m., with the lowest occurring in the middle of the night (2:00 to 4:00 a.m.), while melatonin levels start to rise in the evening and peak between 2:00 and 4:00 a.m. before tapering off into the morning.

Cortisol and melatonin have far-reaching effects throughout the body. If the SCN is the conductor, then it's time for us to meet the musicians sitting on the edge of their seats, attentive to their director: your organs. Nearly every single organ is affected by our circadian rhythm: the intestines, brain, heart, liver, kidneys, lungs, skin, adrenal glands, ovaries, testes, prostate, esophagus, spleen, and thymus. This means our circadian rhythm influences our gastrointestinal, cardiovascular, hormonal, renal, and musculoskeletal systems.

Why Babies Don't Sleep for Four Months

Parents! Have you ever noticed that newborn babies have absolutely no semblance of respect for day and night boundaries? Of course you have. You spent many hours up in the middle of the night, soothing and feeding your baby. Babies are born without a circadian rhythm. In fact, they're not capable of having a circadian rhythm at first. Cortisol comes on board sometime after two months. Melatonin joins the party at three months. Then it takes until four months for things to settle into a pattern. Hopefully by four months you were able to get some sleep!

Your Immune System Is Nocturnal

But what about the immune system? Both melatonin and cortisol play crucial roles in regulating it, ensuring that immune activity aligns with our natural circadian rhythm. This may surprise you, but let's start here: Your immune system is nocturnal—it is more active and does its most important work while you sleep. As melatonin levels rise, you fall asleep but your immune system wakes up. Melatonin enhances the immune system's ability to fight infections, repair tissues, and process immune memory—a key part of long-term immune function. Most importantly, nighttime is when the immune system trains and refines itself, ensuring that it remains well regulated. This makes a ton of sense from an evolutionary perspective. If the immune system were highly active during the day, it would interfere with our ability to think, move, and function—because inflammation, a natural by-product of immune activation, is closely linked to fatigue. To prevent this, the immune system has evolved to be primarily active at night, governed by melatonin to take advantage of the time that we are resting.

This is where cortisol comes in—the yang to melatonin's yin. Cortisol, released by our adrenal glands during the day, is anti-inflammatory and immune-suppressing. It keeps immune activity in check, preventing unnecessary inflammation so we can focus on the demands of wakefulness. Ironically, cortisol functions like melatonin—but in reverse—for the immune system. Just as melatonin signals the immune system to activate at night, cortisol signals it to rest during the day. This daytime reprieve is essential, giving the immune system time to regulate itself and avoid excessive inflammation, which could otherwise lead to autoimmune dysfunction or chronic disease.

Cortisol in balance is a normal, healthy part of our circadian rhythm. Yet we also release cortisol out of rhythm during times of stress. In fact, it is often referred to as our "stress hormone" for this reason. When the body perceives a threat—which could be physical, psychological, environmental, or nutritional stressors—the adrenal glands flood the system with cortisol. Cortisol releases sugar, protein, and fat to make energy available; raises blood pressure; enhances alertness and cognitive function; and suppresses the immune system, digestion, and reproduction. We call this "fight or flight," part of the sympathetic nervous system.

Although cortisol is anti-inflammatory when it's released during the normal ebb and flow of our circadian rhythm, it becomes inflammatory when it's chronically elevated. As a result, the immune system gets dysregulated by not being allowed the opportunity to enjoy a low cortisol period. An extra burst of cortisol is exactly what we would need if we were cave people evading a saber-toothed tiger, but it is not what we need in the middle of the night when we're trying to sleep, since stress causes insomnia. It's not what we need when 88 percent of Americans are metabolically unhealthy and excess stress promotes increased appetite, weight gain, insulin resistance, high blood fats, and high blood pressure—otherwise known as metabolic syndrome. And it's not what we need when dealing with chronic inflammatory conditions, since we know that during high melatonin–low cortisol phases our body fortifies the immune system. Chronic stress is an immune destroyer, which we'll dive deeper into in Chapter 8. For now, the point I'm making is that the rhythmic balance of melatonin and cortisol is central to the optimum functioning of our immune system in part because of the anti-inflammatory properties of daytime cortisol and in part because our nocturnal immune system uses the nighttime to refine itself and learn. As you can see, both cortisol and melatonin are extremely important to our biorhythm.

So how do we get this symphony playing beautifully synchronized music? It should come as no surprise that we accomplish this through our gut microbiome. Much as they play a central role in educating and empowering our immune system, our gut microbes play a central role in our circadian rhythm.

Why You Get Congested at Night

Your immune system has a circadian rhythm, and it's more inflammatory at night. Ever notice that your seasonal allergies and nasal congestion get worse at night? That's proof. Similarly, people with rheumatoid arthritis experience pain and stiffening of their joints overnight and improvement during the day. People with complex inflammatory conditions like Crohn's disease often report worsening symptoms at night, and these symptoms may be dismissed by their doctor. It's real. Your immune system is more active at night.

Dawn and Dusk in the Gut

Your gut microbes, much like you and me, are subject to daily rhythms. Maybe for them it's not the rise and fall of the sun. They don't have a retina or the ability to perceive light. Heck, they live in the crypts of our intestines. But there are other daily rhythms that shape their world, much like the sun shapes ours. For them, it's what you eat, when you eat it, when you sleep and for how long, when you move and how hard, your stress levels, and the timing of prebiotics and probiotics and other supplements and medicines. These factors shape their environment, which shapes the gut ecosystem. You might notice that the things that shape your microbiome are all things that *you* have control over. Timing is everything, and you're setting the clock. Researchers have found that *more than half* of our gut microbial species have their own twenty-four-hour rhythm. The microbes themselves change throughout this cycle, and so does their function. In both mice and humans, the microbiome was observed adapting to a daily routine, optimizing to perform specific functions at specific times. In human studies, the microbiome was focused on energy metabolism and protein production during the day and detoxification at night. Much like our immune system, our microbes literally rise and fall during a twenty-four-hour cycle to help us perform better, sparking our metabolism by day and cleaning up the mess by night.

How connected are your microbiome's daily rhythms with your circadian rhythm? The best way to answer this is to totally disrupt the circadian rhythm and see how much harm it causes. Researchers examined humans flying from the United States to Israel, an eight- to ten-hour time zone shift. They checked the microbiome at specific points—before travel, when the travelers were jet lagged (one day after travel), and when they recovered (two weeks later). Jet lag resulted in dysbiosis and more microbes connected to obesity and metabolic disease. The researchers transplanted the jet-lagged human microbiome into mice, and the mice gained more weight, accumulated more body fat, and spiked their blood sugar. But when the circadian rhythm was restored, so was the microbiome.

There's also evidence that our gut barrier operates on a circadian rhythm. Circadian disruption damages the tight junctions that hold the gut barrier together, resulting in increased intestinal permeability and inflammation. This is why shift workers have higher levels of inflammation in their blood work compared to daytime workers. They have more lipopolysaccharide leaking across the gut barrier.

Interestingly, cortisol is the crucial factor that aligns the gut microbes with the gut barrier, while melatonin has been shown to increase the production of tight junction proteins that fortify the gut barrier. So while our circadian rhythm involves all these factors—when we wake and when we sleep, what we eat/drink/swallow and when—it all ultimately comes back to cortisol and melatonin. Remember, your circadian rhythm is a symphony conducted by the SCN, and our immune system and gut barrier are the instruments.

So when we're talking about healing our immune system, gut barrier, and microbes and lowering inflammation, realigning our circadian rhythm is one of the most powerful levers we can pull. When we wake and when we sleep. What we eat, drink, and when. Let's start with the most powerful of circadian levers—*light*.

The Sun: Nature's Prednisone

If we want your gut microbes and your gut barrier to align with your inner clock, we need to firmly time-stamp the clock and make it totally clear when the day begins and when the day ends. We do this by hacking cortisol and melatonin with light.

Your eye provides the power of vision. The world is made up of different wavelengths of light that represent different colors. When you fix your gaze on something, that spectrum of light enters the eye and gets focused on the retina, and the brain decodes it so you can see.

The SCN is tapping into this information with a singular focus—the intensity of blue light. Blue wavelengths are naturally abundant in sunlight, particularly in the morning and midday. So by focusing on the intensity of blue light, the SCN evolved to detect and align the body's natural rhythms with the rise of the sun.

This makes sense, particularly when you consider that for 99.99 percent of human history, we lived a nomadic lifestyle, using natural shelters like caves and temporary huts. Imagine camping your entire life. When you're camping, you know exactly when the sun rises. There's no missing it. But of course, things changed ten thousand years ago when we transitioned into permanent dwellings and formed settled communities. Even then, the home was a place to return to at the end of the day, but the world in which humans interacted existed outside the home.

It wasn't until very recently, the last few hundred years, that humans moved nearly their entire lives indoors. During the Industrial

Revolution, working on the land was replaced by working in a factory or office. Jobs became concentrated in cities, resulting in urbanization. Electricity and artificial light made us less dependent on sunlight. Planes, trains, and automobiles cut down on outdoor travel. Television, video games, the internet, and TikTok gave us reasons to plop on the couch for hours on end. And then the pandemic gave us "work from home." If you don't have to leave your home for work, you don't even get the time it takes to walk from your house to your car and your car to your office. Now you're just permanently inside. On average, 93 percent of our time is inside.

We have gained a lot. We have also lost a lot. One of the things we've lost is our circadian rhythm. We evolved with the sun and are designed to receive sunlight on a daily basis and align our biology with it. If you're not exposed to the sun, then your body ends up a rudderless ship, and there are consequences to this.

What happens when blue light strikes the retina in the morning hours of the day? First, it cuts off melatonin production. Immediately, cortisol levels increase. With appropriate light exposure, this cortisol lift can be 50 percent or more. As we've discussed, this shift away from melatonin to cortisol enhances alertness, focus, and faster reaction times. Basically, it turns your brain on. It also helps turn your gut on. Cortisol stimulates gut motility. It also shifts our immune system from the pro-inflammatory recovery phase of the night to the anti-inflammatory get-up-and-go phase of the day.

Morning light exposure triggers more than just cortisol release. It also gets serotonin, the "happy hormone," flowing. You've probably heard of seasonal affective disorder, where spending too much time indoors makes people feel depressed. There are innumerable studies showing us that light exposure is good for our mood and can even be used to treat depression. But serotonin is more than a mood hormone. It's also a gut motility hormone, helping to get your gut into a rhythm and even produce a vigorous morning bowel movement. And, interestingly, morning serotonin sets you up for great sleep that night because serotonin is the precursor to melatonin. When you make serotonin in the morning, you get more melatonin in the evening.

Did you ever see the movie *Wall-E*? It's a favorite in our family. Wall-E is a robot trying to survive in a dystopian future. The beauty and natural resources of Earth no longer exist, but one thing that remains omnipresent is the sun. It still sets the rhythm for the world, rising in the morning and falling in the evening. The sun is the source of Wall-E's energy. Overnight, his battery drains and he is a disempowered version of himself until he charges back up. It's a struggle to get himself to the sun, he's so slow and weak in the morning. But when those rays hit his solar panel, it is glorious. The energy bar progressively lights up with a crescendoing *beep beep beep*. Fully charged, he's ready to dominate the day.

In the real world, *you* are Wall-E. Your body craves that morning light. You are a shell of yourself until you get it. But when you step outside in the morning and look up to the sky, here comes that energy filling your battery—*beep beep beep*. I want you to feel it. Be intentional. Take notice of what happens with your body when you orient your first hour to the sun. You will feel it.

A study of college students, who we all know are a circadian *disaster*, found that morning light exposure improved multiple aspects of their sleep that night. They fell asleep faster; they had deeper, more efficient sleep; and although they spent less time in bed, they woke up more rested, alert, and energized the following morning. Do you want these things? Deeper, more restful sleep and alert, energized days? The only intervention was morning light exposure.

Research shows that thirty minutes of morning sunlight is sufficient to train your circadian rhythm. Don't have thirty minutes? That's okay. Less may get the job done, too; it's all a matter of where the sun is, how clear the skies are, whether you are wearing glasses, and where you fix your gaze.

Don't be discouraged if you live in Seattle or London. An overcast day still has twice as much light as an office and three times as much light as an indoor space. Outdoor light is a spectrum of wavelengths from the sun, whereas a light bulb is restricted to specific wavelengths. Your SCN was trained to respond to a spectrum, not a hack. Whenever possible, get the real thing, even if it requires bundling up or grabbing an umbrella.

You may not control the weather or the clouds in the sky, but you control the rest. Let's optimize. The best time to get sunlight is within thirty minutes of waking up. Your cortisol peaks in the first hour, so you want to boost the wave and ride it, not miss it. When you go out, it's preferred to not wear glasses if possible. At a minimum, make sure they're not sunglasses or blue light blockers, as many new glasses have blue light blocking to protect our eyes from devices. Orient to the east when possible. Don't look directly at the sun. Set your gaze up to the sky; observe the tops of trees or where buildings scrape the sky. Enjoy the majesty of blue or the puffy cotton clouds.

I say this to you as I sit here, outside, with my laptop and write this book. You have to be adaptable and possibly creative to get your thirty minutes of morning outdoor time.

Why the Sky Is Blue and the Sun Is Yellow

If sunlight is an abundant source of blue light, why doesn't the sun look blue? Sunlight travels through space before it hits our atmosphere. Blue light has a shorter wavelength, so when it hits our atmosphere, it scatters and spreads, filling out the sky and making it blue. When the blue light scatters away, the sun is revealed as a warm yellow. This explains why the sky stops being blue when the sun sets. The blue sky is literally sunlight. This also means we can give our SCN the blue light it needs by looking to the sky and not the sun.

Circadian Rhythm Impacts Your Gut Rhythm

A great morning bowel movement is the absolute best way to start the day: Am I right? Morning light exposure stimulates cortisol and serotonin release, both of which stimulate gut motility and help to get your bowels into a rhythm. Unfortunately, if you have digestive health conditions like irritable bowel syndrome or chronic constipation, you may have abnormally low morning cortisol levels, indicative of a disrupted circadian rhythm. What we are learning in this chapter is much more than establishing a rhythm to improve your gut or your immune system. This is an opportunity to get your gut in rhythm, too. As a gastroenterologist, I believe that circadian alignment should be part of treatment for all gut motility disorders.

Eat, Fast, Heal, Repeat: Aligning Mealtimes with Your Circadian Rhythm

What we eat, when we eat, and when we choose to *not* eat are all reflected in our microbiome. You and your gut microbes have different needs and abilities at certain times of the day, and there is strong evidence showing us that *when* we eat matters a lot for our health. Nighttime shift work, otherwise known as work-related circadian disruption, has been associated with obesity, diabetes, irritable bowel syndrome, heart attack, stroke, and multiple forms of cancer, including colorectal, prostate, and breast cancer. Shift work has also been associated with increased risk of autoimmune thyroid disease, rheumatoid arthritis, multiple sclerosis, Crohn's disease, and ulcerative colitis.

God bless our civil servants—nurses, hospital workers, police and emergency workers—and many others who work nighttime shifts to help our society function and thrive. Research has shown that you could feed them literally the exact same food and drink, and because they are shift workers, their body will handle it differently. For example, seven days of moderate red wine consumption resulted in increased gut permeability and inflammation in healthy night workers but not healthy day workers. Similarly, when night shift workers were asked to eat only during daylight hours and to fast at night, even though their job required them to be awake during the night and to sleep during the day, those that only ate while the sun was up had significantly better blood sugar control.

What this research tells us is that you could eat the exact same meal at different times of day and get very different results. Our metabolism is strongest in the morning and weakest in the evening. You have better blood sugar and blood fat control in the morning, and this wanes as the day progresses. This explains why one simple change—shifting most calories to the morning instead of the evening—resulted in lower blood sugar, less insulin release, better insulin sensitivity, less hunger hormone (ghrelin), and lower blood pressure. Shifting calories to the morning also led to greater weight loss and a thinner waist even though the same number of calories were being eaten. Think about this—same number of calories, but different timing, and that changes everything.

One detail from that study that really caught my attention: Women who concentrated their calories in the morning experienced a 33 percent drop in triglycerides, while those who consumed most of their calories at dinner saw their triglycerides increase by 14 percent.

Triglycerides are a type of fat found in your bloodstream. After you eat, any excess calories are converted into triglycerides and stored in fat cells for later energy use. Higher post-meal triglyceride levels correlate with increased cardiovascular risk. Moreover, my colleagues at ZOE found a strong link between inflammation and triglyceride levels—

hour by hour, rising triglycerides signal inflammation, while falling levels indicate an anti-inflammatory state. So the aforementioned study suggests that front-loading our food is anti-inflammatory and may explain why skipping breakfast is often associated with higher inflammation. And remember, it's not just food—alcohol also raises triglyceride levels, further contributing to inflammation.

Let's hold on to the idea that inflammation rises and falls with our blood triglyceride levels and explore its implications. In the ZOE study, triglyceride and inflammation levels rose for four to five hours after eating and remained elevated for six to eight hours—this is dietary inflammation in action. Now consider how this ties into mealtimes: Fasting lowers triglycerides and reduces inflammation, while eating late at night, say at 10:00 p.m., sets the stage for unnecessary nocturnal inflammation. It's no wonder late-night eating is associated with weight gain, high blood pressure, elevated cholesterol, diabetes, and cardiovascular disease.

Just twelve hours of overnight fasting offers beneficial changes to the gut microbiome. Extending the fast a little bit longer may increase diversity within the gut microbiome and reduce inflammatory cytokines. If we think about how triglycerides and inflammation stay elevated for eight hours after eating, then this idea starts to really make sense. We are creating an anti-inflammatory window for our gut microbes.

We call this time-restricted eating, or TRE. It's a daily pattern that creates consistency, and for that reason it reinforces our circadian rhythm around mealtimes, helping to get genes that control recovery and inflammation working for us rather than against us. We often focus on the numbers—as in how many hours you were fasting and how many hours you were eating. But let's not overlook the fact that equally important is *consistent* mealtimes. Irregular eating patterns with varied mealtimes have been associated with obesity, type 2 diabetes, and cardiovascular disease. In my opinion, the unspoken, unheralded benefit of TRE is that it brings attention to mealtimes and helps people to establish consistency.

This can change the way that we feel. At ZOE, I was the medical director for a pretty cool study where we had close to forty thousand people doing TRE for two weeks and logging daily into an app how they felt. We asked them to choose a ten-hour eating window, with at least fourteen hours of fasting each day. Here's what happened to those who really did the fasting: For the first forty-eight hours, their hunger got worse, but it got better day by day. Energy levels and mood both improved. Meanwhile, those that were inconsistent with their TRE routine had lower energy, worse moods, and more hunger. Consistency is key.

We also had 68 percent of people report improvements in bloating during the study. This is particularly interesting because our study population was anyone who wanted to try time-restricted eating, so it was more of a general population and not necessarily focused on those with underlying gut issues. Despite this, two out of three participants experienced less bloating.

Most of our study participants were a bit like Forrest Gump: Just as he kept running, they kept fasting. Out of 37,545 who completed the initial study, 36,231 opted for additional weeks of TRE. Highly popular! The reason for this is readily evident. They *felt better*. The benefits that started in the first two weeks got even better—more energy, better mood, less hunger.

But does TRE reduce inflammation? The results of twenty-five combined studies collectively say "Yes!" The anti-inflammatory effects of TRE actually appear to be most powerfully tied to its ability to help us achieve energy balance.

The human body was designed with specific energy needs, and we wake up every day with a natural drive to fulfill those needs. Hunger was meant to be nature's guide to energy sufficiency. For millions of years we lived with food scarcity. Starvation was a very real threat to human life. So we developed hunger cues intending to motivate us to seek energy. This naturally protects us because when we need more energy, we are intrinsically motivated to get it. Starvation puts stress on the body, which activates inflammation. Believe it or not, inflammation helps during starvation because it creates insulin resistance, the same physiology that underpins type 2 diabetes. If you're starving, insulin resistance helps your body raise your blood sugar to maintain energy for the brain. Think about that: The physiology that we associate with obesity and type 2 diabetes actually evolved to protect our brain during times of starvation. We call this antagonistic pleiotropy. The traits that we evolved to protect us end up harming us when our environment changes.

Understatement of the year: A lot has changed since the time when we were cave people navigating food scarcity. Our modern food environment has an unlimited supply, has relatively low cost, requires no effort, and has been designed to hack our brains and make us addicted. Our hunger hormones that signal us to eat when we're starving are also designed to tell us to stop when we've had enough. But hyper-palatable, ultra-processed foods confuse our hunger signals so that we don't actually know if we're hungry or full. Our confusion results in us mindlessly eating without a clear motivation. Simultaneously, our ultra-processed foods put us in an unnatural position where we can radically and consistently overeat, something that would be very difficult to do if you were only consuming whole foods, let alone needed to put in tremendous effort to obtain those foods. The result of consistent energy overconsumption is weight gain, and eventually obesity.

Whether a person is underweight or overweight, energy imbalance always puts a stress on the body that activates inflammation. But when they get back into balance, which means weight gain for some and weight loss for others, there are actually anti-inflammatory health effects. This is because our gut microbiome mirrors what's happening with our bodies on the outside. Being underweight and being over-weight are both associated with a loss of diversity, but when you restore balance, you can actually restore diversity to the microbiome.

Time-restricted eating is a framework to help people achieve energy balance. Body mass index, or BMI, is an imperfect measure of energy balance, but according to the Centers for Disease Control and Prevention, nearly 75 percent of Americans are overweight or obese. Being more precise, 88 percent of Americans are metabolically unhealthy. For these people, there is potential benefit to restoring energy balance.

TRE can contribute to less inflammation because research shows that people are able to achieve calorie restriction, lose weight, recalibrate energy balance, and sustain it with TRE without counting calories. This is particularly interesting because calorie deficit (which promotes energy balance when there's too much energy) has been shown to improve gut barrier integrity.

A recent clinical trial made the national news because it was the first ever randomized controlled trial to show that calorie restriction slows aging. For decades, we thought that our genes were a rigid code for a lifetime of health and disease, but we have since discovered that our genes are actually modifiable thanks to our gut microbiome. This challenges the paradigm that your age is the number of years since your birth and instead suggests that aging is also modifiable, something you can control. Researchers were unsure of why calorie restriction had this effect on aging. I believe the reason is because of the impact that energy balance has on the microbiome, gut barrier, and inflammation.

In the protocol in Chapter 9, we'll walk through how to add TRE to your life in greater detail. For now, consider bringing a more consistent rhythm to your mealtimes. Can you eat your last calorie before 8:00 p.m. and your first fourteen hours later? Try to get the majority of your meals—and particularly the heavier ones—earlier in the day. Notice if you find yourself eating at very inconsistent times or if you have a good natural rhythm already established.

Weight-Loss Drugs: Are We Solving the Right Problem?

As we've discussed, ultra-processed foods hijack our biology, causing us to overeat and disrupting the natural function of our hunger hormones. So how did we respond to this crisis? We created expensive drugs to turn hunger off. In other words, our food system created the epidemic, and now we're trying to fix it with pharmaceuticals. Does that make sense to you? To me, it's like letting a faucet run until a sink overflows, then endlessly mopping the floor instead of just turning off the tap. And let's be real—the pharmaceutical industry profits from keeping that faucet running because they're selling the mops. These drugs are *expensive* and they're generally recommended to be taken *for life*. That's a perfect formula for profits.

Now, don't get me wrong—there are absolutely people who need these drugs. For those with morbid obesity, severe metabolic disease, or high cardiovascular risk, these medications can be life-changing. For these individuals, weight-loss options range from diet and lifestyle interventions to bariatric surgery and endoscopic procedures—and now these medications have been added to that list. For people who really need them, especially when they don't have other options, I'm so glad that we have them.

But that doesn't mean they should be the first-line treatment for everyone carrying extra weight, and they certainly shouldn't be used for vanity purposes. Yet I've heard some people claim that everyone should be on them, justifying it with arguments that they reduce heart disease and may lower obesity-related cancer risk.

This is patently false. The benefits of these drugs—such as reduced cardiovascular disease risk—are applicable only in the populations that they've studied, people with obesity and other health conditions. That's a far cry from saying that someone who wants to lose ten pounds for spring break should microdose them under the illusion of added health benefits.

And let's not ignore the downsides. First, the weight comes roaring back when people stop taking the drug. So if you want to keep the weight off, you may be committing to taking this drug for the rest of your days. That's a big commitment! What if you're twenty years old? Are you going to take this for the next sixty years? Not to be a wet blanket, but we don't yet know the long-term risks beyond the first few years. We'll find out in real time as people take them. People who are signing up now will be our test group.

As a medical doctor, I would be highly cautious before ever making a lifelong commitment to a drug. Make no mistake: All medications carry risks, even the ones that we think are super safe—at some point we realize they weren't. I much prefer a strategy where pharmaceuticals are used temporarily to achieve a specific goal, and otherwise we focus on addressing root causes. The root cause of obesity isn't a lack of GLP-1 drugs—it's a broken food system, metabolic dysfunction, and lifestyle factors that no prescription can truly fix.

If you're looking for something that does address the root of the issue and also protects against heart disease and cancer and more, might I suggest something far safer, far less expensive, that we have far more experience with and evidence for: dietary fiber. If we acknowledge that 95 percent of America is deficient in fiber, it feels like this would be a great place for us to start, and the amount of healing that would occur in this country if we all committed to this would be incredible.

Bottom line: I recommend these drugs only when they're truly needed. For most people, a diet and lifestyle approach is still the best, safest, and most sustainable path to weight loss and long-term health.

You Can Enhance the Benefits of TRE with Exercise

Both time-restricted fasting and exercise improve metabolic health and promote energy balance. Both also enhance gut microbiome health and are anti-inflammatory. And both can be anchored to your twenty-four-hour clock and contribute to circadian health. Of course, timing matters here as well. I'm a big fan of light morning exercise, ideally outside. It helps to activate our metabolism, boost our energy, elevate our mood, and improve our sleep. I don't know about you, but I *need* these things.

As for heavier exercise, my favorite time is late afternoon, around 3:00 p.m. to 6:00 p.m. This is when your body's performance naturally peaks thanks to warmer core temperature, optimized muscle function, and improved coordination, aligning perfectly with your circadian rhythm. Alternatively, fasted morning exercise can enhance fat burning, improve insulin sensitivity, and reinforce circadian alignment by clearly signaling the start of your day.

Of course, there are many factors that we might consider in deciding when to exercise—weather, our personal schedule, and our preferences, which may be informed by our circadian rhythm. Ultimately, finding the ideal time for exercise is intuitive. Experiment with different exercises and different times. Listen to your body. Let it tell you what works best for you. My one request is that you not do heavy exercise late in the evening, as this activates the sympathetic nervous system and can negatively affect your ability to quickly fall asleep.

Sleep: Nature's Recovery Aid

Sleep is a primitive and circadian daily ritual that we share with one another and with our ancestors who evolved before us. But much like how modern life has disrupted our natural eating patterns and hunger mechanisms, so too have we disrupted our natural sleep patterns. And there are consequences to this.

Sleep is powerfully intertwined with inflammation and the health of your immune system. In mice, sleep deprivation accelerates autoimmune antibody formation. In humans, sleep disturbance activates inflammation throughout the body. Perhaps that explains why people have a 70 percent greater risk of developing an autoimmune disease if they have insomnia or why those who sleep less than seven hours per night are more likely to develop lupus. Less than seven hours of sleep per night is also associated with greater risk for heart disease, obesity, type 2 diabetes, and cognitive disorders. But when done properly, sleep is a longevity tool.

A good night's rest is one of the absolute best things you can do for your body. Sometimes I feel like we receive information like this and we don't even process it. Maybe it's because we all *know* that sleep is important. Because it is obvious, it gets glossed over and it's not as attractive as the shiny new toy. But we must truly see this and acknowledge this important fact. Read that last paragraph one more time. Sleep is *central* to our health.

Of course, there are microbiome connections that play a role in the power of sleep. When you have a bad night's rest or inadequate sleep, what do you crave the next day? Carbs! Sugar and flour. Check this out . . . In one study, researchers forced normal-weight men to stay up until 2:45 a.m. and wake up at 7:00 a.m. After just two nights, their microbiome shifted to resemble the pattern found in obesity and they developed insulin resistance. This would result in more insulin release, and insulin levels have been connected to more hunger and craving for simple carbohydrates. In another study, insomnia was associated with a compromised gut barrier. Bottom line: Poor sleep impacts our gut microbiome.

Our microbes aren't just responsive. They play a central role in our sleep. Researchers recently discovered that there are specific bacteria—Selenomonadales and Negativicutes—that promote insomnia. Alternatively Lachnospiraceae and *Odoribacter* are bacteria that promote sweet, restful sleep. Naturally, you're wondering how to get more of the sleepy-time bacteria. The answer is fiber. Fiber has been associated with the microbes that promote better sleep. This was confirmed in a randomized controlled trial where eating more fiber-rich foods resulted in deeper, more restorative sleep, while adding sugar and saturated fat was associated with lighter, less restorative sleep. And then we wonder why so many of us have trouble sleeping.

Gut microbiome diversity has been found to predict multiple measures of sleep quality. A triangular link exists between the gut microbiome, inflammation, and sleep, meaning that when you improve one, you improve the others, and when you harm one, you harm the others. It can be a vicious cycle or it can be a health-boosting feedback loop, depending on which direction you have the triangle moving.

One way to improve your sleep is through increasing your body's production of melatonin, your natural sleepy-time hormone. We can do this through two different pathways. The first is through the brain. I mentioned earlier that melatonin is produced through the transformation of serotonin. The happy hormone becomes the sleepy hormone. This happens in the pineal gland, a pea-size gland near the center of your brain in close proximity to the SCN, where melatonin is both made and released. When we get our morning light exposure, we're filling our brain with the happy hormone. This partially explains why during darker, colder months with less outdoor light exposure, we are more vulnerable to seasonal affective disorder, or a depressed mood. But morning light exposure also provides the brain with the serotonin it needs to make sleepy-time melatonin in twelve to sixteen hours.

As we have learned throughout this chapter, the timing of light exposure during our day is perhaps the most powerful lever that we control for circadian optimization. Much as we should seek unfiltered light exposure in the morning, we should minimize it in the evening. Evening light exposure, especially from artificial sources like screens and LED bulbs, disrupts melatonin release by the pineal gland. The blue light signals to the brain that it's still daytime, suppressing melatonin production and delaying the onset of sleep. This misalignment with our natural circadian rhythm can lead to difficulty falling asleep, poor sleep quality, and increased risk of metabolic and mood disorders.

The melatonin released by the pineal gland is the most tied to our circadian rhythm, but we do have another source of serotonin that produces melatonin and—you guessed it—it's in our gut. Your gut microbes and the intestinal lining cells have the enzymes to create melatonin. It's been well documented that 90 to 95 percent of serotonin is produced in the gut. But did you know that four hundred times more melatonin is produced in the gut compared to the pineal gland? Four hundred times!

What's all that melatonin doing there? First up, gut melatonin promotes a healthy microbiome. It promotes the growth of beneficial species like *Akkermansia*, *Bifidobacterium*, and *Lactobacillus* and has been associated with increased gut diversity. Interestingly, it also helps promote the short-chain-fatty-acid-producing bacteria Ruminococcaceae and *Coprococcus*. We know what happens when we get more SCFAs! For one, they help repair and restore the gut barrier. But they're not the only things that help, because gut barrier cells have melatonin receptors and increase barrier repair proteins in response to more melatonin, as mentioned earlier. When melatonin levels go up, gut permeability goes down.

Immune cells have melatonin receptors, too. Melatonin has a direct impact on numerous immune cells—neutrophils, B cells, T cells, and monocytes. This makes the immune system stronger and more targeted. When you add this to the effects of melatonin repairing the gut barrier, you are creating an anti-inflammatory gut. Beyond bolstering the immune system, gut melatonin influences intestinal motility, digestive enzyme secretion, and the release of satiety hormones like peptide YY. So yeah, there are some good reasons for us to have a ton of melatonin in the gut.

How do we get more of it? Simple. Create a flood of serotonin and let the body (and the microbes) convert it to melatonin. There are four strategies that you can use to pump up serotonin throughout your body. First, you can take advantage of unfiltered morning sunlight, as we've discussed throughout this chapter. Second, exercise has been shown to increase both brain and gut serotonin. Movement—especially aerobic activities like running, cycling, or even a brisk walk—stimulates the release of tryptophan into the brain, fueling serotonin production. Meanwhile, exercise also enhances gut motility and microbial diversity, supporting serotonin production in the gut. This explains why exercise is associated with better mood, mental clarity, and better sleep, and it relieves constipation. If you combine your morning light time with a brisk walk, you are creating the perfect morning routine to reap these rewards.

The third and fourth strategies to naturally increase serotonin occur in the kitchen. We need to feed the microbes two ingredients: tryptophan and fiber. Tryptophan, one of the nine essential amino acids, is the precursor to serotonin. You've heard of tryptophan because it's found in Thanksgiving turkey and gets blamed for everyone falling asleep after the meal. Is the tryptophan in turkey even the cause? Most likely not, actually! (*Mythbusters* strikes again!) The post-Thanksgiving fatigue is probably due to carb overload from the stuffing, rolls, potatoes, and pie. Or it's the booze. Okay, it's both. That said, tryptophan *is indeed* the precursor to serotonin, but also gut microbes produce short-chain fatty acids from fiber, and the SCFAs stimulate the production of serotonin by intestinal cells. So if we want more gut serotonin, I'd suggest eating foods high in both tryptophan *and* fiber. You'll find them concentrated in many seeds and nuts—hempseeds, chia seeds, flaxseeds, and pumpkin seeds as well as walnuts, cashews, and pistachios. When you think of tryptophan, stop thinking of turkey and start thinking of seeds and nuts. They can be a great addition to your breakfast after you take a brisk morning walk.

The name of the game is consistency. So if we want to improve our circadian health, we need to develop consistency around bedtime. This is what most of us refer to as an evening routine. Get your morning light and minimize nighttime light exposure. Get your fiber and your tryptophan and focus on consistency with your bedtime. For more tips on optimizing your sleep environment, check out page 376 in the Appendix.

Creating Your Personal Routine for Circadian Health

Intentional routines are how we build consistency. Establishing a strong, reliable morning and evening rhythm around light exposure, meal timing, and bedtime practices sets the stage for optimal bodily function. By focusing on these "bookends" of the day, you harness the power of the environment and your choices to ride the daily circadian wave. This alignment supports your microbes, immune system, and overall well-being, allowing them to work in harmony with your life goals.

As we close this chapter, consider Melinda's journey. Restoring her circadian rhythm was a pivotal step in managing her ulcerative colitis, illustrating the profound impact of consistency on healing. Her story is a testament to how orchestrating daily routines—prioritizing morning light, structured meals, and consistent sleep—can transform health outcomes.

But circadian optimization is only the beginning. Our exploration of timing has revealed how intricately linked our routines are with our gut and immune health. Now I invite you to dive even deeper. In the next chapter, we'll explore not just *which* supplements support your rhythms and resilience, but *when* to take them—unlocking the power of circadian supplementation.

Chapter 6 is backed by 194 references gathered through an extensive review of the scientific literature. You can browse the full citation list at www .theguthealthmd.com/plantpoweredplus.

CHAPTER 7

OPTIMIZATION

The Art of Strategic Supplementation

There is absolutely no doubt in my mind that supplements can and should be a part of how you achieve better health. But I want to be totally clear on the very first page of this chapter:

They aren't a replacement for healthy food.

They aren't a replacement for a healthy lifestyle.

And they aren't a replacement for the appropriate use of medicine.

Nor are they the same as food, lifestyle, or medicine. They have their own role within your pursuit of optimal health.

I feel like I've been bombarded by extremes when it comes to supplements. On one side, conventional medicine relies heavily on pills and procedures—generally overlooking diet, lifestyle, and supplements altogether. On the other, some dietary zealots treat their nutrition plan like a magic bullet, outlawing any use of supplements or medicines and shaming anyone who dares to use them. Then there are anti-medicine practitioners who prescribe labyrinthine supplement regimens instead of a single, evidence-based drug. And let's not forget the agenda-driven internet voices who criticize supplements as unregulated and unproven but simultaneously see no issue with the ten thousand additives in our food supply that are less regulated and less proven. If you're tired of the insanity and just want to be healthier, I have good news for you. You're in the right place. Let's stop with the games and focus on results—powering your health using whatever works best.

You can't rely solely on nutrition, lifestyle, supplements, or medicine and expect optimal results—overemphasizing one at the expense of others leaves valuable tools on the sideline. The truth is that food, lifestyle, medications, and supplements all offer tremendous potential benefits; and they can work beautifully together. When thoughtfully combined, they create a synergy that can profoundly support your gut health. Think of them all as tools within a four-part framework:

1. **DIET: FOUNDATION.** Aim for a wider variety of plant-based foods, focusing on fiber, polyphenols, healthy fats, and fermented foods.

2. **LIFESTYLE: FORTIFICATION.** Prioritize consistent sleep, movement, stress balance, and emotional and spiritual connection.

3. **MEDICINE: INTERVENTION.** Use evidence-based therapies when needed, guided by your doctor, while still seeking and addressing the root cause.

4. **SUPPLEMENTS: OPTIMIZATION.** Address deficiencies and elevate key nutrients to strive toward A-plus health without being satisfied with a passing grade.

This book is designed to help you get the fundamentals right. We're not here to eat every healthy food in existence, to chase every supplement on the market, or to live the perfect life. But we want to nail the most important stuff.

In this chapter, I'll walk you through the key supplements that support your gut microbiome, help rebuild and repair your gut barrier, and ultimately optimize your immune system to reduce inflammation. But as with all the advice in this book, I recommend discussing any changes with your health care practitioner—their role is to understand your individual health needs and help tailor the best approach for you.

Revisiting Prebiotics, Probiotics, and Postbiotics

In my first book, *Fiber Fueled*, I introduced an important formula:

PREBIOTICS + PROBIOTICS = POSTBIOTICS

Prebiotics are food for your healthy gut microbes. Probiotics are the microbes that provide said health benefits. And postbiotics are what the healthy gut microbes create when you provide them with prebiotics.

Think of the most amazing restaurant. The professional chef—your healthy gut microbes, or native probiotics—uses unique skills to create something extraordinary. But a chef can't conjure a meal from thin air; she needs high-quality ingredients. These are prebiotics. Once she has the right ingredients, she does what she's trained to do: She crafts the most delicious meal, that is, the beneficial postbiotics produced by your gut.

What truly matters is the meal itself—that's what you experience and value. Yet behind every great dish, there's a skilled chef and premium ingredients. Similarly, in your gut, neither prebiotics nor probiotics are effective alone. It's the postbiotics like butyrate, acetate, and propionate that become active and exert biological effects.

Ultimately, our health strategy revolves around this formula. We build a dietary strategy with this in mind—targeting more prebiotics (fiber, resistant starch, polyphenols, healthy fats) and more probiotics (fermented foods). When combined, these create a bounty of postbiotics (SCFAs, bioactive polyphenols, enzymes, healthy fats and peptides, and more). This is why we build our diet around the four workhorses as our foundation.

Yet, 95 percent of Americans are deficient in fiber intake. Eighty to 90 percent of Americans don't consume enough high polyphenol fruits and vegetables. Saturated fat and omega-6s are the dominant fats in our diet, not omega-3s and monounsaturated fats. And fermented food intake is largely nonexistent, as we've replaced our ferments with artificial preservatives and ultra-processed foods. This is the opposite of what it needs to be. It's no coincidence that we have gut and inflammation problems in the United States. People aren't eating prebiotic and probiotic foods.

This is not an argument to supplement our way out of the problem. As I said, food is our foundation. We start by prioritizing fiber, polyphenols, healthy fats, and fermented foods. But there is absolutely room for supplements to make sure that we are getting an appropriate amount of prebiotics and probiotics.

Prebiotics: Your Daily Essential

I have witnessed firsthand the power of prebiotic supplements. I started to use prebiotic fiber supplements in my clinic in 2014 to treat digestive health problems such as constipation, diarrhea, bloating, irritable bowel syndrome, acid reflux, inflammatory bowel disease, and more.

Time and again, I saw patients experience life-changing improvements in their gut health, and the pattern was too consistent to ignore. This isn't surprising when you consider that most people are fiber deficient. When you provide fiber, you are feeding a starving microbial community that's eager to thrive. The result? Your microbes respond with enthusiasm—improving gut health, reducing symptoms, and often creating a ripple effect that enhances overall well-being.

The evidence backs this up. Here are some of the benefits that we've seen in studies with prebiotic fiber supplementation:

- Growth of SCFA-producing gut microbes like *Akkermansia*, *Bifidobacterium*, and *Faecalibacterium prausnitzii*
- Reduced counts of unhealthy microbes such as *Bacteroides intestinalis*, *Bacteroides vulgatus*, and *Propionibacterium*
- Increased short-chain fatty acid production
- Improved gut barrier function
- Reduced bacterial endotoxin levels
- Reduced inflammatory markers like C-reactive protein, interleukin-6, and tumor necrosis factor
- Enhanced immune function
- Improved gut motility
- Less visceral sensitivity
- Improvement of *both* diarrhea and constipation
- Improvements in irritable bowel syndrome symptoms
- Better diabetes and blood sugar control
- Improvements in blood lipid parameters
- Less fat mass and less visceral fat
- Natural increase in satiety hormones GLP-1 and peptide YY
- Suppression of the hormonal stress response and improved neurotic- or pessimistic-type behavior
- Improved absorption of calcium and magnesium
- Reduced risk of nonalcoholic fatty liver disease
- Improved cognitive performance

Interestingly, the benefits of prebiotic fiber supplements aren't exclusive to those who are fiber-deficient. I've had patients come to me with already diverse, fiber-rich diets, yet they still struggled with persistent gut symptoms like bloating, irregularity, or IBS. When we added targeted prebiotic fiber supplements, the changes were often remarkable. This highlights the unique advantage of fiber supplements: They act as a direct, targeted fuel for gut microbes, bypassing the digestion that whole foods require. Whole foods are, of course, foundational for good health and irreplaceable in their nutrient diversity, but their intact food matrix means the fiber they contain has to be unpacked through digestion before your microbes can benefit. Fiber supplements bypass the prep work, delivering chopped-and-ready prebiotics straight to your gut microbes—like serving gourmet ingredients to master chefs so they can effortlessly whip up their signature, health-boosting dish.

The Issue with Prebiotic Supplements and Constipation

We hear all the time that fiber is the treatment for constipation. Unfortunately, it's much more complex than that. Almost everyone with constipation has bloating as one of their symptoms. The bloating improves when they empty their bowels, meaning they relieve the constipation. For people with mild constipation, the addition of a fiber supplement can mobilize their bowels, relieve the constipation, and improve their symptoms. But for people with moderate or severe constipation, a fiber supplement by itself may not be adequate to get the bowels moving. As a result, the fiber sits in the colon, where the microbes ferment it and produce gas. The result is that this person feels *worse* with a fiber supplement. The solution to this problem is to get the bowels moving first—such as with magnesium, which we discuss below. Once they're moving, add the fiber supplement to help keep them moving. It would also make sense to opt for a low FODMAP fiber supplement, which may still produce gas but will be much more gentle, and to start with a smaller dose and then slowly increase the dose over time.

Prebiotic Supplements: Cheat Sheet

Preferred Prebiotics	**Daily Microbiome Nutrition (DMN) by 38TERA** (low FODMAP; 7 prebiotics, including Solnul-resistant starch and Actazin kiwifruit fiber)
	Acacia fiber (low FODMAP)
	Partially hydrolyzed guar gum (low FODMAP)
	Psyllium (low FODMAP)
	Galacto-oligosaccharides
Starting Dose	Start low (1–2 grams or less) to allow the gut microbes to adapt and minimize side effects.
Target Dose	Depends on the fiber type and what is supported by evidence.
Who Should Not Take Them	No hard contraindications, but some people with SIBO (small intestine bacterial overgrowth), constipation, or severe dysbiosis may need to gently introduce them.
Possible Side Effects	Bloating, gas, and abdominal discomfort.
Tips for Optimization	1. **Start low, go slow.**
	2. **Opt for low FODMAP** if you have a sensitive gut.
	3. **Stay hydrated.**
	4. **More isn't always better.** Sometimes lower doses are better.
	5. **Variety is preferred.** Mono-fibers excessively feed the same bacteria.
	6. **May need to treat constipation first** before adding prebiotics.

Probiotics: Let's Get Targeted and Precise

While prebiotics nourish the microbes already living in your gut, probiotics aim to add new microbes to the mix. It's easy to see why probiotics have become the darlings of the supplement world, receiving all the hype and attention. But is it warranted? Not entirely. The truth is that I generally prefer prebiotics over probiotics. Here's why.

Probiotic capsules can add beneficial microbes to your gut, but if your existing microbes are starving due to a lack of prebiotics, what exactly do you expect those new microbes to do? They need fuel to thrive. A chef with an empty fridge is a waste of talent. On the other hand, when you consume prebiotics, you're feeding your gut's native microbes, addressing fiber deficiency, and creating more beneficial microbes—essentially, creating your own probiotics from within.

Additionally, probiotics come with an inherent issue of personalization. Every gut microbiome is unique. So when you take a probiotic, how can you be sure it will integrate well with the microbes already living in your gut? Maybe it will help, maybe it won't, and maybe it will have no effect at all, whereas with prebiotics there's one thing we can say with certainty: Every single one of us has microbes capable of processing fiber. It may not be the same microbes for all of us, but they're there. By activating that part of your gut microbiome through prebiotic consumption, you make these microbes stronger and more effective.

There's also the issue of colonization. Probiotics don't typically stick around in the long term. This may be due to your native microbes keeping them out or it may be that your diet doesn't align with their needs and thus they arrive, starve, then die. Uplifting, I know. But this is another reason I prefer prebiotics. While probiotics don't tend to stay for the long term, resistant starch has been shown to increase the growth of *Akkermansia muciniphila* by 317 percent and *Bifidobacteria* by 350 percent. These microbes play vital roles: *Akkermansia* strengthens the gut barrier and reduces inflammation, while *Bifidobacteria* produce beneficial SCFAs like butyrate. Similarly, fiber from green kiwis has been shown to increase *Akkermansia* and *Faecalibacterium prausnitzii*, both of which are critical for gut health. Instead of taking an expensive *Akkermansia* probiotic that likely won't colonize, you can feed your native *Akkermansia* with the right prebiotics and make it stronger.

That said, I do think probiotics have a part to play. I've had hundreds of patients benefit from targeted probiotics and have great results. I'm simply saying that prebiotics should usually come first, and when it comes to probiotics we have to be more strategic and tactical.

Smart probiotic use means finding the right strain at the right dose for the right condition, as supported by the medical literature. Remember this, or crack this book back open and look it up every time you're thinking about using a probiotic. For example, in patients with IBS, bloating, and digestive distress, I often recommend *Saccharomyces cerevisiae* at a dose of 500 milligrams/day because it has multiple randomized controlled trials demonstrating its efficacy. Similarly, for antibiotic-associated diarrhea, *Lactobacillus rhamnosus GG* has proven effective in both children and adults.

Examples of Targeted Probiotics for Specific Conditions

INDICATION FOR THE PROBIOTIC	STRAIN (BACTERIA/YEAST)	DOSE
IBS with bloating	*Saccharomyces cerevisiae*	500 milligrams/day
Antibiotic-associated diarrhea	*Saccharomyces boulardii*	500–1000 milligrams/day
Acute diarrhea	*Lactobacillus rhamnosus GG*	10–20 billion CFUs/day
Constipation	*Bifidobacterium lactis* DN-173010	1 billion–10 billion CFUs/day
Ulcerative colitis (remission)	*E. coli* Nissle 1917	10 billion CFUs/day

Postbiotics: Coming Soon!

Some people might wonder why we can't just skip the "fiber meets microbe" romance process that culminates with butyrate and jump straight to butyrate as a supplement. We know that postbiotics are the bioactive compounds produced by your gut microbes when they ferment prebiotics. The short-chain fatty acids—butyrate, acetate, and propionate—are examples of postbiotics. As we know, SCFAs have many health benefits: They strengthen the gut barrier, calm the immune system, and reduce inflammation, among many others.

But SCFAs are just the beginning. Postbiotics encompass a diverse mix of microbe-created products. Heat-killed probiotics are no longer alive, yet they still retain biological activity. For this reason we call them "zombie probiotics," and the advantage is that the zombies are more stable than live probiotics. Other postbiotics include microbial enzymes, transformed polyphenols, and even vitamins like B_{12} and K_2, which are synthesized by gut microbes.

There are indeed postbiotic supplements on the market today, specifically butyrate—and I believe that more will be developed in the future. I'm not a fan of butyrate supplements because when you start with fiber or resistant starch, you know you're providing your gut with SCFAs in the right amount exactly where you need them in the colon. Unfortunately, taking butyrate supplements is not the same. When taken orally, butyrate gets absorbed almost immediately, nowhere close to the colon. Even though I'm the president of the SCFA Fan Club, I haven't embraced butyrate supplements—at least not yet. In the future, if we have high-quality randomized controlled trials demonstrating their effectiveness, I'll immediately be on board. Until then, I'm sticking with the good old-fashioned "fiber meets microbe" and let them produce butyrate naturally in the colon, just as nature intended.

Outside of butyrate, I'm actually extremely enthusiastic about the future potential of postbiotics. It's such a diverse category, and as science advances, they will open new frontiers in gut health therapies. We're just now starting to see the emergence of postbiotic technology in the supplement space, and the best is yet to come. But even as new supplements emerge, the best way to harness the power of postbiotics, by far, is by cultivating a healthy gut microbiome, fueling it with premium fuel, and then trusting your microbes to deliver the postbiotics your body needs.

The *Test, Then Address* Approach

I want to take you beyond adequacy and get you to optimization and that means being in the sweet spot. But how do you know when you're in the sweet spot? After all, this requires precision—not too much, not too little, just the right amount. The answer:

TEST, THEN ADDRESS

Testing lets you know where you stand today, allowing you to refine your plan and create a strategy that moves you toward optimal levels. But testing is only the first step. The real magic happens in how you address what you find. Your results give you a road map to take targeted action and track your progress over time. By knowing where you are today, and where you want to be in the future, you can make informed, intelligent choices with the steps that are needed to get you there. In some cases, that may be through dietary adjustments, but generally the most precise approach will be with supplements.

The *Test, Then Address* strategy is a universal approach to targeted supplementation. By identifying deficiencies or suboptimal levels, we can address specific needs with precision. But this strategy also comes with a word of caution: Supplements are powerful tools, and over-supplementing can cause harm. Our goal is not to achieve "perfect" blood work. If you do enough tests, you will always find something that's wrong. The goal is better gut and immune health, not a cluttered medicine cabinet. Don't lose sight of that. Yes, I believe in supplements. But no, I don't believe in taking a hundred of them. As blood work and wearable technology become more pervasively used, I don't want you to get sidetracked trying to perfect everything. Start with this question: "How do I feel?" Because at the end of the day, your well-being is what truly matters. Use supplements that help you feel better.

Targeted Gut-Immune Supplementation: Vitamin D and Omega-3s

Two supplements that are particularly relevant to gut-immune health where we really want to nail the optimization are vitamin D and omega-3 fats.

Vitamin D

Vitamin D isn't just a vitamin—it's more akin to a hormone. Levels fluctuate throughout the day, and it travels throughout the body to target specific cells, binds to a receptor, and activates a physiologic response. Most vitamin D is produced in your skin when exposed to sunlight, hence the fluctuating levels. Specifically, it is ultraviolet B rays from the sun that convert cholesterol into an inactive form. From the skin, it is activated in the liver and kidneys before binding to receptors found in nearly every tissue in your body: in your gut (where it strengthens the gut barrier), in your immune cells (where it regulates inflammation), and in bones, muscles, and even the brain. Its far-reaching effects make vitamin D a critical player in health.

Research has demonstrated its pivotal role in autoimmune disease, gut health, and immunity. For instance, the VITAL trial was a nationwide study where twenty-five thousand generally healthy adults over age fifty took 2,000 IU of vitamin D daily for an average of five years. In that study, they found that vitamin D supplementation reduced the risk of autoimmune disease by 22 percent. Importantly, these were not high-risk people. In theory, new autoimmune diagnoses should be *rare*. So to achieve a 22 percent reduction in *all* autoimmune disease incidence is profound. Many people who are healthy and well want to know, "What's one thing I can do to protect myself from developing an autoimmune disease?" Here you have your answer.

But that's just one study and there are many more. Another study showed that vitamin D supplementation increased gut microbial diversity, a key marker of a healthy microbiome. In patients with inflammatory bowel disease (IBD), vitamin D supplementation improved clinical symptoms and intestinal inflammation. This goes along with a meta-analysis of eighteen randomized controlled trials involving 908 patients showing that vitamin D supplementation protected inflammatory bowel disease patients from relapse.

Whenever possible, it makes sense to *Test, Then Address* with vitamin D. This allows you to know where you stand and to fine-tune so you can hit the sweet spot. The preferred test is 25-hydroxyvitamin D, which reflects your body's vitamin D status. Levels below 20 ng/mL indicate deficiency, but aiming for 30–50 ng/mL is optimal for most people. For those with autoimmune conditions, targeting 40–60 ng/mL may yield additional benefits.

Vitamin D Supplements: Cheat Sheet

Dose	**Maintenance Dose:** 1,000–2,000 IU/day for general health.
	Deficiency Correction: 4,000–5,000 IU/day, with monitoring.
	High-Dose Therapy: 50,000 IU weekly for severe deficiency under medical supervision.
Test, Then Address	Measure 25-hydroxyvitamin D in the blood.
	Healthy Individuals: 30–50 ng/mL
	Inflammatory Conditions: 40–60 ng/mL
Who Should Not Take	Hypercalcemia (sarcoid, hyperparathyroidism, etc.), kidney disease
Possible Side Effects	Rare, but hypercalcemia, kidney stones, calcification of tissues
Tips for Optimization	1. **Take with healthy fat.** Vitamin D is fat-soluble, so it's absorbed better with fat.
	2. **Consider sun exposure.** This is one of the benefits of spending time outdoors. Of course, we must avoid sunburn and use sunscreen strategically. There is variability by skin type, season, and time of day. A UV index of 3 or higher is required for vitamin D production.

Omega-3 Fats

Omega-3 fatty acids—specifically EPA (eicosapentaenoic acid) and DHA (docosahexaenoic acid)—are powerful anti-inflammatory agents with a unique ability to influence gut and immune health. Unlike the shorter-chain omega-3 ALA (alpha-linolenic acid) found in flaxseeds, chia seeds, hempseeds, and basil seeds, EPA and DHA come primarily from marine sources like algae and fish and are directly utilized by the body. DHA, in particular, plays a critical role in gut health by supporting the intestinal barrier and fostering beneficial bacteria. Unfortunately, the conversion of ALA to EPA and DHA is inefficient—less than 5 percent in most people. So it makes sense to source EPA and DHA either in our diet or in supplement form.

Studies show that EPA and DHA supplementation can reduce inflammation, improve gut microbial diversity, and support the immune system. For example, omega-3 supplementation has been shown to increase SCFA-producing bacteria and provide health benefits, leading scientists to now argue that omega-3 supplements are in fact prebiotic.

A moment ago, we discussed the VITAL trial with vitamin D. But that wasn't just a vitamin D trial. Omega-3s were included in that study as well, and researchers found that when 1,000 milligrams per day of DHA and EPA omega-3 supplementation were included along with vitamin D, the risk of autoimmune disease dropped by roughly a third.

Much like with vitamin D, omega-3 supplementation is an opportunity to *Test, Then Address*. The omega-3 index, which measures the EPA and DHA levels in your red blood cells, is how you do it. A level below 4 percent is considered deficient, while an ideal range is 8 to 12 percent. For those with chronic inflammatory conditions, optimizing omega-3 levels through diet and supplements can be a game changer.

Omega-3 Supplements: Cheat Sheet

Dose	**General health:** 500 milligrams/day of combined EPA and DHA. **Inflammatory conditions:** 1,000–3,000 milligrams/day of combined EPA and DHA.
Test, Then Address	Omega-3 index (percentage of EPA and DHA in red blood cell membranes) **General health:** 8–12 percent **Inflammatory conditions:** 10–12 percent
Who Should Not Take	Bleeding disorders, on anticoagulants, allergies, those at risk for atrial fibrillation
Possible Side Effects	Fishy aftertaste or belches, nausea, loose stool, increased bleeding
Tips for Optimization	1. **Choose high-quality sources.** Free of heavy metals, PCBs, and other contaminants. 2. **Consider algae-based.** Straight from the source, fewer contaminants, more sustainable. 3. **Take with meals.** Enhances absorption and reduces side effects. 4. **Reduce competing fats.** Minimize omega-6 fats found in seed oils to create better balance between omega-6s and omega-3s.

Circadian Supplementation: Melatonin, Magnesium, and Zinc

As we learned in Chapter 6, our bodies operate on a natural rhythm that impacts everything from our sleep-wake cycles to hormonal fluctuations and even when we poop. Hopefully while reading that chapter you were taken aback by how powerful and how pervasive circadian rhythms are. They're there, and you can either ignore them and struggle against the current or acknowledge them and let them propel you. Supplements are an opportunity to align with this rhythm.

To keep it simple, we should split our supplementation protocol in two—morning and evening. This allows us to take our daytime-fueling supplements in the morning and our rest and recover supplements in the evening and build consistency, which we know is the key to optimizing our circadian health. The supplements we've discussed so far— prebiotics, vitamin D, and omega-3s—fit naturally into a morning routine, as they align with daytime activity and metabolic processes. Now it's time to fill in our evening supplement routine with melatonin, magnesium, and zinc.

Melatonin

In Chapter 6 we discussed melatonin, the "sleep hormone," which sets our rest and recovery rhythm at night, in the darkness. Melatonin is naturally in the pineal gland and even more so in the gut, and its secretion increases in response to darkness, signaling the body to wind down for rest. Supplementing with melatonin can improve sleep onset and quality to enhance our nighttime circadian rhythm. But there's an opportunity for supplementation to simultaneously improve our sleep and our gut-immune health. In Chapter 6, we discussed that melatonin is good for the microbes, the gut barrier, and the immune system and also influences motility and digestion. With that in mind, there are clinical trials supporting the use of melatonin at night to improve irritable bowel syndrome, acid reflux, ulcerative colitis, and healing intestinal ulcers. Importantly, we should start with a low dose and gradually increase it because if we overshoot, you'll end up groggy the following morning.

Melatonin Supplements: Cheat Sheet

Dose	General use: 0.5–3 milligrams/day for sleep and circadian rhythm.
	Higher dose: 5–10 milligrams/day for conditions that require more.
Test, Then Address	No specific target level is established.
Who Should Not Take	Pregnant or breastfeeding (not studied)
Possible Side Effects	Drowsiness

Tips for Optimization	1. **Timing matters.** Take 60 to 90 minutes before bedtime.
	2. **Start low and go slow.** If you overshoot, you'll be drowsy in the morning. Ease into dosing to find the lowest effective dose.
	3. **Optimize your environment.** This means reducing evening light exposure, particularly from devices, which will disrupt your body's natural melatonin production.
	4. **Pump your morning serotonin up.** Serotonin produced in the morning becomes melatonin in the evening. In Chapter 6, we discussed four strategies to accomplish this—unfiltered morning sunlight, exercise, fiber, and tryptophan-rich foods.

Magnesium and Zinc

Magnesium and zinc are complementary to melatonin. Magnesium amplifies the effect of GABA, which is a neurotransmitter that has a calming effect on the brain and contributes to sleep. By the way, this is also why magnesium is helpful for anxiety and migraine headaches. Meanwhile, zinc contributes to sleep by supporting neurotransmitter function and contributing to melatonin production.

While melatonin, magnesium, and zinc are celebrated for their sleep-enhancing properties, in this chapter we're supplementing to optimize our gut-immune health, so let's look at what they do there. As we learned in Chapter 6, melatonin promotes the growth of beneficial gut bacteria, increases gut barrier repair proteins, and regulates several immune cells. Magnesium's benefits for gut-immune health are similarly impressive. Magnesium also supports the gut barrier and improves the function of immune cells, enhancing the body's ability to fight infections and control inflammation. This explains why magnesium supplementation significantly reduces C-reactive protein levels.

Meanwhile with zinc, I think of gut barrier repair. Back in 2006, I was an intern (first year after medical school) at Northwestern in Chicago and we would use zinc supplements and lactulose, a prebiotic, to treat hepatic encephalopathy—a brain dysfunction where toxins in the blood from cirrhosis and liver dysfunction cause confusion and altered consciousness. I knew back then that the brain and liver were involved, but it wasn't until ten years later that I realized that what we were *really* treating was a damaged gut barrier. Along these lines, there was a 2001 study called "Zinc Supplementation Tightens 'Leaky Gut' in Crohn's Disease," and more recent evidence has also suggested benefit for rheumatoid arthritis. It's worth noting that zinc also plays an important role in wound healing and collagen production.

When it comes to supplementation, not all forms of magnesium and zinc are created equal. Magnesium glycinate is the best choice for improving sleep, as it is highly bioavailable and less likely to cause digestive upset. For those seeking to address constipation, magnesium oxide and magnesium citrate are better options, as they have a mild laxative effect. Zinc can be tough on the stomach, so it's often best taken with food to reduce nausea. Zinc picolinate and zinc citrate are two forms with good absorption rates and tolerability.

When possible, we want to *Test, Then Address*. While severe deficiencies are uncommon, subtle imbalances can affect health. Serum magnesium levels should ideally fall between 1.7 and 2.2 milligrams/dL, while zinc levels are best maintained between 70 and 120 µg/dL. Regular monitoring, particularly when supplementing in the long term, is essential to avoid oversupplementation. High doses of zinc, for instance, can interfere with copper absorption and should not be taken in excess for extended periods.

Magnesium Supplements: Cheat Sheet

Dose	Elemental magnesium refers to the actual amount of magnesium in a supplement. For example, 400 milligrams of magnesium oxide contains 240 milligrams of elemental magnesium.
	General health: 200–400 milligrams/day of elemental magnesium.
	Therapeutic dose: Up to 600 milligrams/day, particularly for conditions like migraines, anxiety, or constipation, under medical supervision.
Test, Then Address	**Healthy individual:** 1.7–2.2 milligrams/dL
	Inflammatory condition: Aim for the upper end of the above range.

Who Should Not Take	Kidney disease, heart block, low blood pressure
Possible Side Effects	Diarrhea, cramping, low blood pressure, myasthenia gravis
Tips for Optimization	1. **Choose the right form.** See below. 2. **Take in the evening for better sleep.** 3. **Be wary of the laxative effect.** This will help those with constipation but may loosen up bowels for those that don't. Fiber supplementation or combining magnesium with a calcium supplement can help to address this.

Zinc Supplements: Cheat Sheet

Dose	**General health:** 8–11 milligrams/day of elemental zinc. **Therapeutic dose:** 20–40 milligrams/day of elemental zinc for short-term use.
Test, Then Address	**Healthy individual:** Serum zinc levels of 70–120 µg/dL. **Inflammatory condition:** Aim for the upper end of the above range.
Who Should Not Take	Hemochromatosis, stomach ulcers
Possible Side Effects	Nausea, vomiting, abdominal discomfort, metallic taste, copper deficiency
Tips for Optimization	1. **Choose the right form.** See below. 2. **Take with food.** 3. **Be careful not to oversupplement in the long term.**

Choosing the Right Forms of Magnesium and Zinc

VARIETY OF MAGNESIUM	PREFERRED USE	VARIETY OF ZINC	QUALITIES
Magnesium citrate	constipation, depression	**Zinc gluconate**	mild taste, moderate absorption
Magnesium glycinate	anxiety, relaxation, sleep	**Zinc picolinate**	high absorption, well tolerated
Magnesium malate	fibromyalgia, chronic fatigue	**Zinc sulfate**	low absorption, harsh taste, gastrointestinal side effects

Magnesium oxide	constipation, acid reflux	Zinc citrate	mild taste, moderate absorption, well tolerated
Magnesium threonate	mental clarity	Zinc oxide	low absorption, often used on skin

Curcumin: Nature's Anti-Inflammatory Drug

My dad was a massive guy: He was six feet, seven inches tall and had a size fifteen shoe. It was fun watching him play basketball, but it wasn't fun trying to shoot over him as a kid. Anyway, later in life my dad had really bad knees. He probably needed knee replacements but was trying hard to avoid it, which resulted in his taking huge doses of ibuprofen—three pills, four times per day—to control the pain. When I caught wind of this, my heart skipped a beat. As a gastroenterologist, I'd spent my days (and too many nights) fighting the negative effects of nonsteroidal anti-inflammatory drugs (NSAIDs)—stomach ulcers, bleeding intestines, inflamed colons, and failing kidneys. I told him immediately, "Dad, you need to start taking turmeric." I put him on a protocol of daily turmeric use in combination with black pepper. More on that in a minute. Anyway, it did the trick. My dad's ibuprofen use went from twelve pills per day down to occasional use, as needed. That's a huge win for health, and I'll tell you why.

Turmeric, the vibrant yellow spice derived from the root of *Curcuma longa*, has a rich history in Ayurveda and Chinese medicine. The secret to turmeric's health benefits lies in its active compound, curcumin, a polyphenol with uniquely powerful anti-inflammatory and antioxidant properties. Today, science is catching up to what ancient traditions understood intuitively: Turmeric is a potent tool for supporting health, especially in managing inflammation.

Curcumin works by targeting the same inflammatory pathways as NSAIDs, such as blocking cyclooxygenase-2 (COX-2) enzymes to reduce pro-inflammatory compounds like prostaglandins. Additionally, curcumin inhibits nuclear factor-kappa B (NF-κB), a central regulator of inflammation, and reduces levels of pro-inflammatory cytokines like tumor necrosis factor alpha (TNF-α) and interleukin-6 (IL-6). But the beautiful thing is that curcumin achieves these effects with a very different risk/benefit ratio than pharmaceuticals. Rather than conferring substantial risk without much benefit, turmeric is offering many benefits with limited risks.

It starts with the effects of curcumin on the gut microbiome. Studies show that curcumin promotes the growth of beneficial bacteria such as *Bifidobacterium* and *Lactobacillus,* the SCFA producers that help us to repair and restore the gut barrier. At the same time, curcumin suppresses pathogenic bacteria that can drive low-grade inflammation. This dual action—enhancing beneficial microbes while reducing harmful ones—strengthens the gut barrier, improves microbial diversity, and lowers systemic inflammation. Research has highlighted curcumin's ability to mitigate dysbiosis and fortify the gut barrier, making it a tool that we can use to fortify our gut-immune health.

Turmeric's anti-inflammatory activity translates into tangible health benefits for a variety of inflammatory conditions. In arthritis, curcumin has been shown to reduce pain and improve joint function, rivaling the efficacy of NSAIDs without the associated risks. That one's for you, Dad! A smaller study found curcumin to be superior to an NSAID for rheumatoid arthritis. For inflammatory bowel disease, curcumin has been found to decrease symptoms and oxidative stress, making it a valuable adjunct for conditions like Crohn's disease and ulcerative colitis. Likewise, irritable bowel syndrome shows improvement in symptoms with turmeric. Metabolic syndrome, another inflammation-driven condition, also benefits from turmeric, with improvements in markers such as insulin sensitivity, lipid profiles, and inflammatory mediators. Moreover, its systemic effects extend to cardiovascular health, where curcumin improves vascular function and reduces oxidative damage, which is the opposite of what you find with NSAIDs. Mood disorders such as depression have also shown improvement with curcumin, likely due to its role in reducing neuroinflammation and supporting brain health.

One of the challenges with curcumin is its low bioavailability, meaning the body has difficulty absorbing and utilizing it effectively. Remember what we learned in Chapter 5 about polyphenols—they're big molecules and hard for the body to absorb. However, strategies exist to overcome this hurdle. Combining curcumin with black pepper, which contains piperine, can enhance its absorption by up to 2,000 percent (!!!) by inhibiting the enzymes that break it down.

Consuming curcumin with healthy fats, such as those from avocado or olive oil, also improves its bioavailability, as curcumin is fat-soluble. Additionally, combining curcumin with minerals like magnesium and zinc can further stabilize it and enhance its uptake. Thus, consider taking your morning turmeric/black pepper and your omega-3 and vitamin D supplements with some fat, and take your evening turmeric with your sleepy-time minerals. These approaches ensure that curcumin delivers its full benefits to the body. Taken in the morning, it provides anti-inflammatory support that helps the body stay resilient throughout the day. Taken in the evening, turmeric promotes relaxation and supports healthy sleep patterns, making it a valuable addition to any nighttime routine. Its dual role in supporting both daytime and nighttime health underscores its unique and versatile value as a supplement.

Turmeric and curcumin are both ancient remedies and scientifically validated tools for modern health challenges. Their ability to reduce inflammation, support gut health, and address a variety of inflammatory conditions makes them a cornerstone of a proactive health strategy, while practical strategies to enhance absorption ensure that their benefits are fully realized. For anyone seeking a natural and effective way to combat inflammation, turmeric stands out as a golden opportunity.

Turmeric/Curcumin Supplements: Cheat Sheet

Dose	**General health:** 500–1,000 milligrams/day of curcumin extract (standardized to 95 percent curcuminoids). **Therapeutic dose:** Up to 2,000 milligrams/day of curcumin extract, divided into 2–3 doses, under medical supervision.
Test, Then Address	No specific target for curcumin monitoring has been established.
Who Should Not Take	Gallbladder issues, bleeding disorder, pregnancy, abnormal liver tests from supplements
Possible Side Effects	Digestive issues, low blood pressure, poor iron absorption, abnormal liver tests at high doses
Tips for Optimization	1. **Choose high-quality supplements.** Ninety-five percent curcuminoids, third-party tested for purity and safety. 2. **Combine with black pepper or healthy fat.** Increase absorption. 3. **Take in the morning with omega-3s and vitamin D for anti-inflammatory benefits.** Choose this option if inflammation is worse during the day for you. 4. **Take in the evening for relaxation and gut repair.** Choose this option if inflammation is worse for you at night.

My Approach to Strategic Supplementation

Supplements are a way to optimize the nutrients that matter most to your gut-immune health. This isn't a comprehensive list—additional supplements may be relevant to your unique needs and health history. If I were working with you individually, I'd create an individualized plan for you. In my absence, it's best to consult with a qualified health professional.

When selecting supplements, always let scientific evidence be your compass. If you're considering prebiotics, for instance, seek out a blend that includes multiple fiber types, resistant starch, and polyphenols—because, as we've learned, diversity is key to nourishing a wide range of gut microbes. Make sure that each ingredient has research backing its benefits and that any claims are science-based. Finally, I'm a strong proponent of low FODMAP prebiotics because they are more gentle, cause less bloating, and are just as effective and impactful. (For specific product recommendations, visit theguthealthmd.com.)

Beyond an evidence-based formula, it's crucial to look for rigorous quality standards. Choose products with a clear and complete ingredients list containing high-quality ingredients that are backed by research. Proprietary, trademarked ingredients usually undergo independent testing and often have clinical research to ensure safety, purity, and efficacy. Avoid supplements with artificial colors, flavors, preservatives, and other additives that are harmful to the microbiome. Make sure your supplements are produced under high manufacturing standards, such as Good Manufacturing Practices (GMP) and accreditation by FDA (United States), FSANZ (Australia, New Zealand), or other global regulatory standards. Perhaps most importantly, they should be third-party tested to guard against contaminants like heavy metals, pesticides, harmful microbes, allergens, food intolerance triggers, or banned substances. Frankly, I'd trust a well-tested non-organic product over an untested organic option every time. Organic implies safety, but testing confirms it.

When we implement supplements, there are a few important concepts that I want you to keep in mind. First, it's best to add one supplement at a time, whenever possible. It's nice to know what is doing what. By adding one thing at a time, you'll be able to tell whether it's helping, hurting, or doing nothing at all.

Second, it's often necessary to ease into things. Whether it's prebiotics, omega-3s, melatonin, or turmeric, there is such a thing as too much and too fast. I've taught you to start low and go slow when it comes to your diet. This is also true for our supplements. Your body needs time to adjust, and rushing the process can lead to discomfort or side effects that might discourage you from continuing. Starting low and going slow allows your body to adapt naturally.

And third, make sure to keep the concept of circadian supplementation in mind. Timing is everything. It's easiest to split your day in half, and then fit in your supplements and get consistent with how you take them. In a perfect world, set a daily timer.

Last but not least, don't take supplements just because you heard they were good for you. You should take supplements because they make a difference in your life. Either you feel the difference, or you are optimizing your blood work or you are growing beneficial bacteria in your microbiome. The point being, if you use a supplement for a period of time and you can't tell the difference, it's time to start asking whether you actually need that supplement.

About My Company—38TERA

As a gastroenterologist, I've always held my patients' health to the highest standard. Yet, when it came to recommending supplements, I often felt stuck. I couldn't find products that met my rigorous expectations for quality, safety, and efficacy. For years, I made do with what was available, but deep down, I knew we could do better— much better. That's why, after three years of development behind the scenes, I launched my gut health supplement company, 38TERA, in 2024.

The name "Tera" means trillion, and 38TERA represents the thirty-eight trillion microbes living inside our gut—a thriving community at the heart of our health. Every decision in developing these products has been rooted in science, my clinical experience, and a relentless commitment to creating something that truly works.

On a personal level, building 38TERA has been one of the most fulfilling journeys of my life. Everything that I create—including books, courses, and supplements—is about giving you the tools you need for healing. Combining my passion for clinical care, research, and education with product innovation has been deeply rewarding. Every time someone reaches out to share how 38TERA has improved their health, I'm reminded why I started this in the first place: to make a difference in people's lives and help them achieve their health goals. Developing these products isn't just about creating supplements—it's about challenging the mediocrity in the industry and raising the bar for gut health.

That said, this chapter isn't about 38TERA—it's about you. Whether or not you use 38TERA products, my ultimate goal is to empower you to create a diet, lifestyle, and supplementation protocol that helps you thrive and crush your health goals because, at the end of the day, your health is what matters most.

Beyond Supplements: Your Next Steps

In this chapter, we've explored the core principles of supplementation—everything from testing and correcting deficiencies, to selecting evidence-based, quality products, to aligning them with your circadian rhythm. These guidelines form the bedrock of a smarter, more strategic approach to supporting your gut-immune health.

But let's not forget the bigger picture: Health is more than just diet, lifestyle, and supplements. Emotional and spiritual well-being play a huge role in healing, too. In the next chapter, we'll shift our focus to the powerful connections between trauma, emotional resilience, spiritual health, and your gut-immune system. This holistic lens—body, mind, and spirit—is what truly unlocks your body's full potential. I can't wait to show you what's next.

Chapter 7 is backed by 113 references gathered through an extensive review of the scientific literature. You can browse the full citation list at www .theguthealthmd.com/plantpoweredplus.

CHAPTER 8

BODY AND MIND HEALING
Nourishing the Soul Through Connection

Throughout my career I've had dozens of patients whom even my best medicine failed. I had the perfect plan, the right drugs, the nutrition, sleep, exercise, and other lifestyle factors locked in. Over the course of multiple visits we progressed in our plan, but it just wasn't working. For some patients, it can feel like they've hit a dead end and it's time to find a new doctor.

But often we've just hit the line that exists between the body and the mind. We've reached the furthest limit of what we can do to heal the physical body, and we must now step into the realm of the nonconscious mind and the core self. Unfortunately, most doctors are not trained to do this. Doctors are taught that there is a diagnosis and a pill or a procedure to treat it. That would work if we were just a physical edifice. But we are so much more. We have a mind that conjures thoughts, memories, and emotions and processes information in ways that are both apparent in our conscious mind, and shrouded, implicit, and behind the scenes in our nonconscious mind. We also have a soul, which is the essence of who we are. It gives us purpose, meaning, and connection to something greater than ourselves. This is our core self.

My goal with each patient is to identify the root of their illness and address it. Sometimes our illnesses originate in our physical bodies, and sometimes our physical symptoms come from unwellness in our minds and souls—the relationship between them is intertwined. So far I've covered nutrition and lifestyle changes, but that's not where our journey to heal your immune system by way of your gut ends. I want to take you beyond the body and into the opportunity for healing that exists in the mind and soul because in my experience, that's often where the greatest opportunity for healing exists.

I first learned this in 2010 when I was—reluctantly—assigned to work in the clinic of Dr. Douglass Drossman, Professor of Medicine and Psychiatry at the University of North Carolina. Interesting combination, right? Medicine *and* psychiatry. Dr. Drossman is a pioneer in gastroenterology, known for founding the Rome Foundation and advancing our understanding of IBS through the mind-body connection, emphasizing holistic care that addresses both physical and psychological aspects of gut disorders. Without a doubt, his work has transformed the way we diagnose and treat IBS, making him an internationally recognized leader in functional GI medicine.

In his clinic I had the opportunity, for the first time, to see that there was a world beyond for healing the physical body when we focus on the nonconscious mind and the core self. In Dr. Drossman's clinic, we spent multiple hours with every patient. This was partly because people were flying internationally to see us and partly to facilitate accelerated bonding and maturation of the doctor–patient relationship so that we could discuss sensitive issues like chronic pain, mental health, interpersonal relationships, childhood experiences, trauma, and abuse. I worked with many patients during this time who showed me the power of the mind, soul, and body connections within the gut and the immune system.

In that clinic I witnessed transformations that were borderline miraculous and that went beyond traditional medicine. I saw patients who had spent years trapped in cycles of chronic pain, digestive distress, and autoimmune flare-ups finally break free—not just through medications but through deep emotional work and a reconnection to their core selves. Lifelong conditions that had defied conventional treatment began to shift as we addressed the underlying trauma, stress, and subconscious patterns driving their symptoms. It was healing at the deepest level, where mind, body, and gut came together in ways that modern medicine rarely acknowledges.

As I sat in that clinic, witnessing profound healing unfold before me, I began to see my own story with greater clarity. Each time a patient unloaded bottled-up emotions, frustrations, and past struggles, I couldn't help but think that I should be the one in that seat. As I've shared in my other books, this was a time in my life when I was struggling deeply—with gut issues, food intolerances, weight gain, metabolic dysfunction, anxiety, depression, and crushingly low self-esteem. Changing my diet was essential for improving my health. But in order to truly be well and thriving, I needed to address other issues. Working in Dr. Drossman's clinic opened my mind in ways I hadn't expected. I began to revisit my own childhood, uncovering and processing experiences that were still shaping me in ways I hadn't fully understood. I realized that to truly heal, I had to look beyond what I was eating and address what I was holding on to.

In the conventional medical model, my digestive and mental health struggles would be treated as separate and distinct issues by a gastroenterologist and psychiatrist. But this fragmented approach overlooks a fundamental truth: The gut and brain are not isolated entities but are deeply intertwined through what we call the gut-brain axis. The hours upon hours I spent day after day with my patients at this clinic made it increasingly clear to me that there was more going on for me than just "physical health issues" that were separate from "mental health issues."

Your Two Nervous Systems

You won't be surprised to learn that one central way your physical and mental health is connected is through your gut—by way of your gut-brain axis. This is all thanks to your enteric nervous system. You've probably heard a lot about your central nervous system, which is what we classically think of when we think of the nervous system—your brain and your spinal cord. But you are actually blessed with two separate and distinct nervous systems. You also have an enteric nervous system, a network of five hundred million neurons embedded in the walls of the gastrointestinal tract that controls essential digestive functions such as peristalsis (the movement of food through the gut), secretion of enzymes, and regulation of blood flow within the digestive system. *Five hundred million!* That's five times the number of nerves that you'll find in your spinal cord.

A network of nerves is what we call a nervous system. On a simple level, nerves allow us to measure our inner state and the outer world and then orchestrate an appropriate response. These nerves gather information through our senses—sight, hearing, smell, taste, and touch—and then enact responses through muscles contracting or relaxing or by triggering the release of hormones or neurotransmitters that change bodily function.

If we zoomed in with a microscope, we'd see that the five hundred million neurons lining the gastrointestinal tract are positioned right next to the immune system, which is densely concentrated just beyond the gut barrier—and neither is far from the gut microbes. In the Introduction, I described the gut microbes and immune system as neighbors. But now imagine them living together on a cul-de-sac with your gut nerves—so close that if you peeked out your window, you'd see them all right there, influencing each other in real time. For better or worse, physical proximity results in overlap and connections. When microbes and immune cells release cytokines, your nerves can sense this is happening. Inflammation in the gut actually changes the nerves. We see this in irritable bowel syndrome when people develop hypersensitivity of their gut. The five hundred million nerves in the gut are feeling and sensing and then sending that information up to the brain. They also coordinate different aspects of digestive function, and for this reason we call it the "second brain."

Why have two nervous systems? It's evolution, baby. Over millions of years our enteric nervous system evolved first, allowing increasingly complex life to get access to nutrients through digestion and to fortify defenses through the immune system. We may call it the second brain, but from an evolutionary perspective it's the other way around. The enteric nervous system was your "first brain."

Think about it: You can't grow a tree without first putting down roots to pull in nutrients. With these foundations in place, the brain was given what it needed to grow and become more complex. And, with the enteric nervous system regulating digestive function, the brain was given the freedom to think without having to devote precious resources to the complexities of digestive function. If you've ever been overworked, then you know that fresh ideas and creative thought need space to develop.

Your gut and your brain are best friends. They are constantly talking to each other. They're like teenage besties who chat on the phone, tag each other on social media, and send direct messages throughout the day. Through multiple forms of communication they're able to stay perpetually connected to each other. They always know where the other one is and what they're up to.

Much like teenagers have their preferred tools for communication, the gut and brain have specific ways that they stay connected to each other. The five hundred million nerves carpeting the gut are constantly feeling and sensing signals that come from the gut microbes or the immune system. Let's make an attempt at understanding the breadth of what we're dealing with here. In your gut there are five hundred million nerves that are feeling and sensing the thirty-eight trillion microbes and 1.3 trillion immune cells that reside in the gut.

That's a whole lot of information right there, where things are dynamically changing by the fraction of a second, and all of it gets funneled into a pair of nerves called the vagus. The vagus has been termed the "wanderer nerve" because of its long path through the body, starting in the brain, leaving through a special channel in the skull, descending through the neck to the heart, lungs, gut, and immune system. This is the information superhighway between the brain and the body.

Most of the vagus nerve—about 80 percent—is used to send signals from the gut to the brain, allowing your brain to sense what's happening there. These are your "gut feelings." Your brain is sensing what's happening in your gut through the vagus nerve. The brain and the gut may seem distant from each other, but courtesy of the vagus nerve, you can think of the brain as being right there, next to the microbes and immune cells, because in a way it is.

There's a lot to feel. Your microbes produce short-chain fatty acids, gut neurotransmitters, and other bioactives. Your gut barrier has enteroendocrine cells that produce various neurotransmitters and hormones including GLP-1, the hormone popularized as weight loss and diabetes drugs. The regular gut barrier cells (called enterocytes) and the immune cells produce cytokines. The end result is a diverse mixture of chemical signals that influence the vagus nerve and thereby have the ability to influence the brain.

There are over thirty neurotransmitters produced in the gut, including 90 to 95 percent of your body's serotonin and 50 percent of its dopamine. While most of these neurotransmitters don't cross into the brain—stopped by the blood–brain barrier, which functions much like the gut barrier with its tight junctions—they can still affect mood and brain function in two key ways. First, precursor molecules that do cross the barrier can transform into neurotransmitters on the other side. Second, gut neurotransmitters can stimulate the vagus nerve, and functional imaging studies show that signals from the gut reach brain regions that impact our emotions, mood, and cognition.

The story is different for short-chain fatty acids. When they approach the blood–brain barrier, it's like being a weary traveler far from home finding a kindred spirit—familiar cell types, tight junctions, and protective functions echoing those of the gut barrier. Much like short-chain fatty acids—specifically butyrate—repair the gut barrier, so too do they repair the blood–brain barrier. It makes sense: The most powerful way to repair the tight junctions in the gut barrier is with butyrate. Why would the tight junctions in the brain be any different?

But it doesn't stop outside the brain. It continues *inside* the brain because SCFAs are able to cross the blood–brain barrier, much like they can cross the gut barrier, and directly influence neurologic function. While this is an area of new and exciting research and we have a lot to learn, thus far we know that SCFAs improve memory and learning; regulate neurotransmitter levels that impact mood, emotion, cognition, and reward; and alter satiety through brain hormones. There may be anti-inflammatory underpinnings to the cognitive perks we get from SCFAs. Research has found that SCFAs actively reduce neuroinflammation within brain tissue—a process thought to contribute to conditions such as depression, Alzheimer's disease, Parkinson's disease, multiple sclerosis, and other neurological disorders.

While I'd like to keep discussing the many ways SCFAs are our steadfast allies, we now must return to our long-standing enemy—lipopolysaccharide. We've learned that LPS normally gains access to our bloodstream by crossing a compromised gut barrier, often referred to as "leaky gut." Although the immune system attempts to intercept it, some LPS still makes it into circulation, triggering systemic inflammation. But what happens when LPS reaches the blood–brain barrier? The answer is a "leaky brain." LPS can compromise the brain's protective barrier, allowing it to cross into brain tissue. This breach brings the inflammatory battle from the gut into the brain, leading to neuroinflammation. In mice, a single shot of LPS is enough to trigger neuroinflammation that alters the brain and cognitive function for ten months. Whoa. LPS and neuroinflammation help explain how dysbiosis deep in the gut can manifest as neurologic disease, affecting mood and cognitive function. While this destructive pathway underscores the peril of a breached barrier, there's another side to the gut-brain connection that operates continually.

Through the vagus nerve, the gut is speaking to the brain, and the brain is listening. But it's also responding. Twenty percent of the fibers in the vagus nerve are for the transmission of information from the brain back down to the gut. Through the vagus nerve, the brain can act as the puppeteer—pulling the strings to control gut motility, our stress response and the release of cortisol, and the immune system in the intestine. Of course, all of these factors have the ability to influence and change the gut microbiome. Additionally, the brain releases a hormone called corticotrophin-releasing hormone, or CRH, which activates our stress response but in the process compromises the gut barrier. This explains why stress increases gut permeability. We touched on this topic in Chapter 6 when we acknowledged that cortisol maintains our daytime rhythm yet becomes inflammatory when it is out of rhythm and chronically elevated.

What emerges from this intricate interplay is a seamless connection among the brain, the gut, and the immune system, all orchestrated by the vagus nerve. The relationship is bidirectional: The brain influences the microbes, and the microbes in turn shape the brain. This dynamic communication network is known as the brain-gut axis, underscoring how deeply intertwined our mental state, gut health, and immune responses truly are.

Life on Overdrive: The Toll of Chronic Stress on Our Gut-Immune Health

The gut-brain axis isn't a new idea. In 1872, the founder of modern evolutionary theory, Charles Darwin, wrote this:

> *When the heart is affected it reacts on the brain; and the state of the brain again reacts through the pneumo-gastric [vagus] nerve on the heart; so that under any excitement there will be much mutual action and reaction between these, the two most important organs of the body.*

As Darwin argues, the vagus nerve plays a role in the autonomic nervous system, which is the body's automatic regulator of our heart rate, breathing pattern, digestion, and stress response. This is one part of the nonconscious mind, in that your brain is controlling this for you independent of your conscious thought. It does this by trying to understand what's happening in the world around you and then optimizing your bodily functions to that. But what happens if the autonomic nervous system is reacting to a threat, a ghost, that doesn't exist?

You may be familiar with the two opposite and antagonistic branches of the autonomic nervous system—the sympathetic and parasympathetic. The sympathetic nervous system is your body pushing the accelerator, charging up the body to deal with stress or danger. When the body feels threatened, it automatically hits the gas. The parasympathetic nervous system is the brake. It's how you rest and digest when you are safe and secure, no longer sensing threat. It allows you to feel comfortable in a social environment.

We evolved to survive not just in safety and comfort, but also in environments that are dangerous and life threatening. We don't want this, obviously, but sometimes that's where we find ourselves. A saber-toothed tiger surprise. Rustling in the bushes and you're all alone. Going to war with the enemy tribe. A near miss in traffic. Hardcore flight turbulence. Accidentally hitting "reply all" when you didn't mean to and not being able to unsend. Through human history, the threats have evolved but the way that our nonconscious mind responds remains the same.

Sometimes we don't need to be in survival mode. Sometimes we would be better off feeling safe, comfortable, and unthreatened and allowing our body to rest, to digest, to heal, and to feel at ease in our relationships with others. Would you agree that the modern world has a heavy foot on the accelerator? Whether it is social media, news meant to trigger, the daily grind, "keeping up with the Joneses," social divide, mistrust of our institutions, financial strain, work-life imbalance, expectations, maintaining an image of perfection . . . I could keep going. What would you add?

Our lives are on overdrive. But when do we ever step on the brake? I tried to create a list of aspects of our culture that help us slow down and engage our parasympathetic nervous system, and what I realized is that our modern way of life has increasingly pushed these things away: taking a walk, holding hands, family dinners, ritual teatime, community celebration, outdoor recreation, prayer, worship, and keeping the Sabbath, storytelling and social entertainment, dances. We call them old-fashioned and discard them, but what if there is wisdom in our old ways?

Our biology remains the same, but our environment has changed. Our modern lives are dominated by the sympathetic, which means stressed, threatened, insecure. Do you ever feel that way? I sure do. If we want to restore balance, it starts with seeing the problem that exists. We are not nourishing our parasympathetic nervous system nearly enough.

This chronically stressful "always on" environment has implications for our gut and immune health. You've probably experienced this. Picture yourself in that moment where you're feeling super stressed about something. Maybe it's a breakup or a fight with someone you love. Maybe it's pressure at work, a big test, or the need to make a big public presentation. How do you feel? For many, their acute stress manifests in their gut. It may start with butterflies in the stomach; then it grows into discomfort that's dull at first, but then waves of discomfort build and come through and it's sharp. This is often accompanied by messed-up poops—either explosive, urgent diarrhea or your bowels clam up and you don't poop for a few days. Gut function can be altered by emotions and stress. These are manifestations of the brain-gut axis.

This can go both ways. I've heard about "gut feelings" since I was a kid in the 1980s. It's a popular term referring to our instinctive feelings or an intuitive hunch without any rational basis. We attribute these instincts to our gut. "I'm going with my gut" is something I've said many times when I make a decision based on my instincts and without the ability to really explain it. And research would suggest that although this may seem reckless, our earliest impressions when confronted with a problem can be more accurate than analyzing it more thoroughly.

Do those gut feelings truly originate in the gut? We don't fully know. What we do know is that your gut, through the vagus nerve and other forms of communication, has the ability to directly impact your emotions, mood, and cognition. It's likely that our gut feelings are evolved instincts involving the rapid consolidation of information from the brain, the nonconscious mind, and the gut to guide a sense or feeling around a decision.

As more research helps us understand the power of the gut-brain connection, and the vagus nerve as their go-between, the vagus nerve has become a target for medical intervention for people suffering with disorders of the brain-gut axis. There's an implanted medical device called a vagus nerve stimulator, which is simply a battery-powered box that delivers an electrical pulse through an electrode to the vagus nerve.

Think of a pacemaker, except rather than connecting to the heart it's connected to the vagus nerve. Although you may be hearing about this for the first time, we've been studying vagus nerve stimulation for a long time and the stimulators are now FDA approved for the treatment of epilepsy, depression, stroke rehabilitation, migraine and cluster headaches, and obesity. There's evidence to suggest that vagus nerve stimulation may also be beneficial in treating Alzheimer's disease, Parkinson's disease, and autism. These disorders are all manifestations on some level of the brain-gut axis.

How does vagus nerve stimulation impact the immune system? Vagus nerve stimulation is anti-inflammatory. One of the ways it reduces inflammation is by repairing and restoring the gut barrier, reducing intestinal permeability and inflammation. It also helps the immune system to contain its response to lipopolysaccharide, effectively cooling off the immune cells that live at the gut barrier and are constantly getting poked by what sneaks across. The result is lower cytokine levels and lower C-reactive protein, indicating less inflammation in the body. With this in mind, there have been successful clinical trials using vagus nerve stimulation to treat inflammatory bowel disease, rheumatoid arthritis, lupus, and systemic sclerosis.

The reality, for better or worse, is that our modern culture and lifestyle are as disconnected from our core self as they are from our ancestral diet and circadian rhythms. Allowing ourselves to float along in modern culture is chronically triggering our sympathetic nervous system, unnecessarily activating our stress response, taking down our gut, and creating inflammation in the process. Much like we need to shift our modern diets and daily routines, we must intentionally support the healthy functioning of our central nervous system. We should consciously identify and reduce aspects of our lives that trigger strong emotions and activate the sympathetic nervous system. More importantly, we need to adopt lifestyle practices that don't just restore balance but actively flip our nervous system toward parasympathetic dominance.

Using Heart Rate Variability to Measure the Speed of Your Autonomic Nervous System

While we may think of our heartbeat as having a specific cadence and rhythm, it turns out that every single beat is at least slightly off rhythm from the last one. We call this the heart rate variability, or HRV, and it reflects the balance between the sympathetic (accelerator) and parasympathetic (brake) branches of your autonomic nervous system. Think of it as a speedometer for your nervous system, showing how well your body shifts between stress and relaxation. We want a high HRV because it indicates greater adaptability and resilience, meaning your body is better able to handle stress and recover. We get a high HRV when we're activating the parasympathetic nervous system. Interestingly, a high HRV has been associated with greater gut microbiome diversity. Conversely, a low HRV suggests chronic stress or poor nervous system regulation and has been associated with inflammation. There are multiple studies where increasing HRV was associated with improvements in IBS symptoms. Measuring HRV is easy with wearable devices like smartwatches, making it a practical tool to track your body's stress response and overall health. We'll come back to HRV in Chapter 9 as we build out our personalized plan.

Techniques to Stimulate the Vagus Nerve

Should we all ask our doctors to implant devices to stimulate our vagus nerve? Heck no! There are simple, noninvasive, and free tools that we can use to activate our vagus nerve and we should all (myself included) be looking to pile these up as much as possible in our lives. More is better, and you will feel the difference!

- Deep breathing exercises
- Cold exposure
- Sauna
- Warm bath
- Meditation and mindfulness
- Yoga and tai chi
- Singing, humming, and chanting
- Laughter
- Massage
- Acupuncture
- Regular physical exercise
- Social connection
- Falling in love
- Quality sleep
- Deep pressure and weighted blankets
- Hugs and romantic kisses
- Holding hands and human touch
- Sexual intimacy
- Prayer and worship
- Positive affirmations and gratitude
- Spiritual music
- Relaxing hobbies
- Spending time in nature

Beyond Stress: Treating Your Gut—and Your Immune System—by Healing Trauma

For some of us, the wounds of our past cut deeper than modern-day stressors, and they may not be as overtly obvious because they are hidden within the depths of our nonconscious mind. What I'm referring to is trauma. For some of you, this will be the most important part of the book.

In Dr. Drossman's clinic, it was part of our standard practice to spend about thirty minutes with the patient, then leave for ten minutes before going back in for another thirty-minute session. It was like squeezing multiple visits into one. It also allowed us to progress into deeper, more sensitive topics because it felt natural to the patient that each session would go a little deeper and into topics that hadn't been previously discussed.

Getting into sensitive topics wasn't just something that happened passively: It was very intentional. These patients had already sought second, third, and fourth opinions before coming to see us. They brought binders filled with all the tests. We'd review it to make sure that nothing was missing, but generally these were people who had every test under the sun done twice over. Repeat testing can make sense when it's been a while and needs to be brought up to date, but it doesn't make sense to follow the same playbook that's failed before. With these patients, it makes more sense to try something different and explore powerful health connections that exist in the nonconscious mind. This means discussing a person's childhood or major life events. In most cases, we would find something, some traumatic event, that perhaps wasn't something they were literally thinking about but was an engine of negative energy running twenty-four hours per day.

I'll never forget one woman who had suffered from debilitating irritable bowel syndrome for over a decade. She had seen countless doctors, tried elimination diets, and taken medications, but nothing provided lasting relief. It wasn't until we started talking about her past that a different story began to emerge. She had endured an abusive relationship in her early twenties, one she had long since left behind yet never fully processed. As we worked through it, something shifted. The more she acknowledged the pain she had suppressed, the more her gut symptoms began to ease. It didn't happen overnight, but with cognitive behavioral therapy (CBT), guided journaling, and emotional processing, her IBS—which had controlled her life for years—began to fade into the background.

As I sat in that clinic and witnessed how addressing and releasing past trauma was allowing people to heal, I couldn't help but question whether my own childhood and life experiences were holding me back. It all started on a random day in second grade when my mom came to pick me up from school. The van was packed to the gills and I had a small designated spot to sit. We left Syracuse, New York, and drove seven hours away to the Jersey shore. Everyone in my family was there, except one person—my dad.

None of this made sense to me at the time. I was seven years old. But over the following months, I had to reconstitute my life in this foreign place, and like it or not, things were different. We were living in someone else's house. I was starting over in some other school with people I didn't know and they didn't know me. We were suddenly very poor. And my dad wasn't there. Things were hard and confusing for a long time. Years of legal and custody battles followed; sessions with child psychologists who would use what I said in court; my mom strained to care for my brothers and me while earning her degree to make a better life for us; and there was a visitation schedule with my dad that disrupted my ability to feel really at home in any one place. Eventually, I cut my dad out of my life altogether. I'll come back to that later.

By working in Dr. Drossman's clinic and seeing others heal by releasing their trauma, I began to understand my own issues. Yes, I needed to improve my diet. I wrote about that in *Fiber Fueled*. But there was an emotional element to the way I ate. Junk food was a form of therapy for a soul that was hurting deep down inside. For most of my adult life, I didn't love myself. I also rejected my dad and chose to not accept the love that he had for me, and I paid the price for this.

Trauma creates wounds that don't simply fade with time. These wounds linger in the nonconscious mind, draining energy and creating a ripple effect throughout the body. And while these experiences may be tucked away—hidden from our daily thoughts—they are not forgotten by the body. Trauma can be a monster that haunts us, one that never sleeps and constantly exerts its influence on our mental, emotional, and physical well-being. Your gut feels it, your immune system senses it, and your health bears the brunt of its weight.

But what is trauma, really? It's easy to think of trauma as only the most dramatic events—an assault, a life-threatening accident, or the horrors of war. But trauma is more nuanced than that. It's any experience that overwhelms our ability to cope, leaving behind emotional and psychological wounds. It's losing a loved one, enduring the pain of divorce, or growing up in an environment of instability. It's moments of neglect, feelings of abandonment, or bearing witness to violence. All will leave wounds in the nonconscious mind, the extent of which depends on the individual and the extent of the trauma.

Traumatic experiences, particularly in early life, can change how your brain and your body work. Trauma primes the amygdala, the brain's "fear center," to become hyperactive and hypervigilant, sending distress signals even in safe settings. The nonconscious mind—responsible for tuning your autonomic nervous system to the world around you—ends up chronically misreading your environment, trapping you in survival mode. The unbalanced autonomic nervous system becomes sympathetic dominant, making it difficult to engage the restorative, parasympathetic state. The body's stress response stays locked in overdrive—like a car with the accelerator pinned to the floor—driving a relentless and excessive surge of corticotrophin-releasing hormone (CRH) through your system.

Excessive CRH has consequences in the gut. There are CRH receptors in the muscle cells of the intestines, which disrupt gut motility. There are CRH receptors in the gut barrier cells, which disrupt tight junctions and result in leaky gut. And there are CRH receptors in the immune cells lining the gut, which stimulate the release of proinflammatory cytokines.

Your gut microbes are surrounded!

They may not have CRH receptors themselves, but when you change gut motility, damage the gut barrier, and activate the inflammatory immune response, you have a setup for dysbiosis. As we know, there are consequences to dysbiosis. Does it surprise you that chronic stress and excessive CRH reduce the populations of short-chain-fatty-acid-producing bacteria like *Faecalibacterium prausnitzii* and *Akkermansia muciniphila*? What this illustrates is that chronic stress—especially the persistent activation of your sympathetic nervous system due to trauma—not only disrupts the gut microbiome and damages the gut barrier but also fuels systemic inflammation. Far from being passive bystanders, our gut microbes actively respond to these stressors, playing a central role in our health and disease.

Via the gut-brain axis, a disrupted gut increases the risk of mood disorders—depression, anxiety, and post-traumatic stress disorder—later in life among those with a history of trauma. Via the gut-immune axis, trauma contributes to more inflammation during adulthood and increased risk for autoimmune diseases including rheumatoid arthritis, inflammatory bowel disease, thyroiditis, lupus, and Sjögren's. Via the gut-metabolism axis, trauma contributes to high blood pressure, abnormal blood lipids, and obesity. But really, everything that I just called out is the consequence of inflammation fueling disease.

Let me show you an example of this in action. Researchers studied children and adolescents who were adopted before age two and compared them to children who were raised by their biological parents without any known early life trauma. Now here's the thing: They were adopted before age two. Do you think they can remember this at all? Not consciously. But the nonconscious mind remembers. The children who were separated from their biological parents had lower gut diversity and more inflammatory bacteria. These children, years later, had more gut symptoms and more anxiety. When researchers studied their brain with functional MRI, they found altered brain activity patterns, particularly in the parts that control emotional functioning. The gut and brain changes were connected.

It's really important that we open our eyes and see that our past informs our present, including our gut, our mood, and our health. If you've never made this connection before, consider this your invitation to start paying attention now. There may be something from your past that bothers you to this day. It hurts to think about, so you tuck it away, hoping that if you ignore it long enough, it will lose its power over you—but deep down, you know it's still there.

This chapter is for you.

The first step to healing is to understand how the past informs our present. The next step is to seek professional help to heal the wound. This is not what I do because I am not a trained psychologist or psychiatrist. But if you were my patient, we would discuss finding someone in your community to assist you with this process. Some of the treatment methods that can help include cognitive behavioral therapy, trauma-focused therapy, eye movement desensitization and reprocessing (EMDR), and cognitive processing therapy, as well as medications when needed.

Not every bad thing that happens is trauma and life is not an endless series of traumas before we die. Thank goodness, because that's a dark and depressing worldview that will make you, well, dark and depressed. It's important to not interpret the world as trauma focused or life as being defined by victimhood. This creates unhealthy patterns of thought that actually activate the CRH and sympathetic response; in other words, they give rise to unnecessary dysbiosis and inflammation.

Life is filled with challenges—and we should embrace them. Confronting and overcoming obstacles makes us more resilient, more confident, and more capable of handling whatever comes next. If you allow challenges to stop you in your tracks, you stunt your growth. If you overcome them, you transform those hurdles into stepping stones that propel you forward. I love the poem "Good Timber" by Douglas Malloch published in 1922, shortly after World War I and the Spanish influenza pandemic took sixteen million lives and fifty million lives, respectively. The world was going through hard times.

Good timber does not grow with ease:
The stronger wind, the stronger trees;
The further sky, the greater length;
The more the storm, the more the strength.

We will all experience hard times in our lives, but you can embrace the value that comes from challenges. Your muscles get stronger with challenges. Your gut gets stronger with challenges. *You* get stronger with challenges.

But we also need to acknowledge that some difficult life experiences do stay with us for longer than we may like, and our immune and gut symptoms may be a sign that our nervous system is in need of some healing. The difference between trauma and stressful events is the lingering effect that trauma has on our brain, stress response, and gut. Everyday challenges, even when stressful, do not have the sustained effect that I have described in this section, whereas true traumas do. Most everyday challenges are obstacles for us to overcome on the spot. With trauma, the obstacle persists until we get the help that we need to close the wound and move forward with our lives. This isn't to say that the trauma disappears. There will always be a scar that persists as a relic of the injury that we absorbed and overcame. The difference is that it no longer causes the same kind of pain.

The Spectrum of Trauma

Acute Trauma	Car accidents, sudden loss of a loved one, physical injury, sexual assault, acts of violence.
Chronic Trauma	Childhood neglect, prolonged emotional or physical abuse, bullying.
Developmental Trauma	Parental divorce, abandonment, or inconsistent caregiving.
Relational Trauma	Betrayal, unhealthy relationships, traumatic breakups.
Life Disruptions	House fires, natural disasters, job loss, or financial ruin.

The Power of Breath

When you're upset, has someone told you to "take a deep breath"? Diaphragmatic breathing, often called belly breathing, is a simple yet powerful technique to calm the mind and body that improves IBS and constipation. Imagine sitting quietly with one hand on your chest and the other on your belly. Slowly inhale through your nose for a count of four, feeling your abdomen expand as your diaphragm engages. Then exhale through your mouth for a count of six, sensing your belly fall and a wave of calm wash over you. This deep breathing activates your parasympathetic nervous system, reduces stress, lowers blood pressure, and improves lung function. Over time, this practice can ease anxiety and clear the mind to rejuvenate the body and spirit. Don't wait until you're stressed to do it, though. Practice it regularly. Make it a part of your morning or evening routine. Consider adding it to mealtimes if you have food intolerances. Just three minutes is a good place to start, working toward ten minutes per day.

The Power of Connection for Emotional and Spiritual Healing

We are all impacted by the power of connection. Just as our body has a natural appetite for food, our soul has an appetite for connection—both human and spiritual. We can ignore those needs, take the chance they go unfulfilled, and suffer the consequences that come from that. Or we can acknowledge our inner appetite for connection, satiate it, and witness the power it has in our gut-brain-immune relationship.

Human Connection

You can't change the fact that we are social creatures who require human connection to thrive. We evolved to be this way. In prehistoric times, human connection was necessary for survival. Our ancestors faced threats from weather, predators, natural disasters, and other humans. We formed into tribes so that we could work together for shared safety, cooperation, and aggregation of resources. The collective whole was stronger than the individual parts. Being cast out—or isolated—was tantamount to death. We grew to trust and depend on one another because that was the only way we could survive.

But these connections were not based on someone clicking a cheesy thumbs-up or swiping right on their phone. They were profound, mutual bonds of trust and loyalty that were earned. You knew, without question, that the people in your circle would protect you, support you, and help you survive when life got tough. If your tribe was attacked, you knew that another person would put their own life on the line to protect yours, and you would be ready to do the same for them.

Our tribes grew to include many people, but they always started with an essential core—family. All humans are born into a family. From birth and through life, the family was the network of unconditional love and security that provided a foundation for confidence, resilience, and growth. Children were invested into and nurtured to adulthood as eventual contributors to the family. There was collective progress and strength through the formation and growth of a family across generations. The strongest tribes were a family of families.

Through our evolutionary history, the measure of success was always to create a large, multigeneration family. This ensured our ability to endure hardships and thrive as a species. As civilizations advanced, we became seduced by new measures of worth—material wealth, individual achievements, and the pursuit of status. Yet no amount of money, fame, or accomplishment can replace the fulfillment and self-worth that come from human connection and mutual support.

When this foundation is absent or broken, we feel vulnerable. We lose the sense of safety and strength that comes from knowing we are loved and supported. This is not just an emotional reality; it's a biological one. Research shows that social isolation and loneliness are linked to depression, anxiety, increased inflammation, and death at a younger age. In fact, the risk of death from social isolation is considered on par with smoking fifteen cigarettes per day or drinking a six-pack of alcohol.

I definitely felt this when I was disconnected from my dad. Deep down inside, I knew that my dad loved me. But I refused to acknowledge it. Instead, I pushed him away, and eventually that choice reached a point of commitment where it was hard to turn back. And it hurt me. I was hurting myself. If I could go back, I would have asked my younger self to find forgiveness.

Our need for connection is reflected in our gut microbiome. We share microbes with those closest to us. In fact, a recent study found that spouses share more microbes with each other than they do with their siblings. This suggests that microbial sharing is more important than how we were raised. Interestingly, this microbial exchange was not driven by shared dietary habits but was closely tied to the strength of their connection. Spouses who reported feeling deeply connected shared more microbes than those who felt less bonded. Moreover, married couples had greater microbiome diversity compared to those who lived alone, with the highest diversity observed in couples who felt strongly connected. Independent of marital status, other research found that as we get more connected to others and feel less lonely, our gut diversity goes up.

Activation of our stress response may explain this. Remember that the activation of the sympathetic nervous system and the release of CRH have consequences in our gut microbiome, gut barrier, and immune system. Isolation is stressful and is known to powerfully activate the sympathetic nervous system and trigger the release of CRH, setting off this cascade of gut-immune disruption.

But on the flip side, why do we hug, kiss, or hold hands? These interpersonal expressions of human connection and bonding have been shown to stimulate the vagus nerve and parasympathetic nervous system for rest and repair. In fact, scientists now believe that the autonomic nervous system plays an essential role in the formation of romantic relationships and partner bonding. And let's not forget that kissing involves the transfer of about eighty million microbes, so they get to play a role as our little matchmakers.

We are magnets for human connection. When a person is taken hostage and is left with the choice of isolation versus forming an emotional bond with their captor, they will choose connection. This is called Stockholm syndrome. You may think that sounds stupid, but it's actually a survival mechanism. Alternatively, solitary confinement is a form of torture, while deliberate exclusion and ostracizing are emotional abuse. But in today's world, most loneliness is not malicious. Instead, it is our culture, lifestyle, and new technology that have caused us to drift so far from our tribal origins that it is incompatible with our need for human connection.

There are two major aspects of Western culture that are making us disconnected. First is individualism, which says that success is defined by our ability to be independent and self-sufficient. We all strive to purchase a home and live a life separate from our parents as a way to prove our adequacy. The second is materialism, which teaches us to define our value and self-worth by the size of our house, the car we drive, the clothing that we wear. There's the added pressure of maintaining the standards of living established by our parents, because to take a step backward would make you a failure by this standard. But the cost of education, the cost of housing, and the cost of living have all disproportionately increased relative to our income. The financial pressure is mounting.

One response is often to work longer hours, dedicating more time and energy to earning a living. Another has been to prioritize career stability and delay marriage and starting a family. For many, it means both parents entering the workforce, leaving less time for nurturing connections at home. Others may choose to have fewer children—or none at all—as the cost of raising a family becomes increasingly burdensome. These adaptations might address financial strain, but they also come with a significant price tag: the erosion of the deep, meaningful connections that have traditionally grounded us and given our lives purpose.

The deeper we sink into a world defined by possessions and social comparisons, the more isolated and unfulfilled we become, highlighting that the essence of our happiness lies not in what we have but in who we are connected to. Truly.

As a society, we have become enamored with ourselves. Narcissism has seeped into the cultural fabric, brought on by our materialism and nurtured by media and technology. It began with the elevation of movie stars and rock legends, people whose fame was celebrated above their substance. But social media has leveled the playing field, where now you don't need to be a movie star or rock legend to be famous. Now anyone can be internet famous if they get enough likes, shares, and followers. All they have to do is post a glamorous, beautiful, perfect version of themselves for others to aspire to. Or they trade dignity and self-respect for attention—selling access to their bodies, fabricating controversy, entertaining like a clown, or exposing their most intimate moments, all for the sake of followers, validation, and quick cash.

Simultaneously, we are addicted to our devices. We spend an average of six hours per day on them. Pretty wild when you consider that these devices didn't exist twenty years ago and now they consume more than a third of our awake time. Much like we've filled our diet with junk food, we've filled our time with digital junk and then complain that we're too busy. That's lost time that you could be spending with another person forming a connection or developing new skills or sleeping or exercising. But instead, we are on our device, and the research says that makes us less productive, more easily distracted, less present with others, and less able to enjoy connections with friends and family. It is also associated with low self-esteem. For example, parents who use their smartphone find it hard to feel connected to their kids and enjoy time with them. As we consider the importance of the bond between parent and child in this chapter, think about how disruptive that is. We may trivialize it, but our device addiction is hurting our kids.

This cultural shift is taking a toll, especially on younger generations. Research has shown that if an adolescent spends more than an hour online per day—just one hour—it starts to have a negative impact on their psychological well-being. That includes "less curiosity, lower self-control, more distractibility, more difficulty making friends, less emotional stability, being more difficult to care for, and inability to finish tasks." The more time they spend, the worse it gets. It's sobering to consider that the average adolescent spends seven hours per day on devices. And it's no coincidence that rates of depression and anxiety among adolescents have increased significantly in recent years, coinciding with increasing screen time and social media use.

The forward-facing camera on our phones, and the "selfie" culture it created, is perhaps the most tangible symbol of our collective narcissism. It's a literal display of self-focus, where we turn the lens on ourselves and seek validation not from meaningful human connections but from fleeting digital interactions. The impact is readily apparent. The rates of depression and anxiety were relatively stable among adolescents until 2011, and then they took off. Boom—skyrocketing. What happened? It was in 2010 that Apple released the forward-facing camera phone.

Social Media Overwhelms Our Ability for Emotional Processing

We weren't designed to manage a network of thousands, constantly exposed to the emotional highs and lows of others as we are through social media. The endless stream of information triggers us in ways that our ancestors never experienced, overwhelming our emotional capacity. Yet, the internet didn't create our disconnection—it arrived in a world already deeply disconnected. Long before social media, many people had already lost their sense of belonging, of being truly seen and valued by *real* people in their *actual* lives. In the tribal communities we evolved from, our social circles were small, intimate, and contained—focused on a limited number of people with whom we shared powerful, meaningful bonds, groups with whom we could establish real, valuable, and healthy esteem and status. By contrast, social media replaces depth with breadth and friends with followers, leaving us overstimulated, offering no real foundation for self-worth. As a result, we're cut off from the genuine relationships we truly need.

Society tells us to "put yourself first," as though self-care and self-comfort are the ultimate solutions to our unhappiness. We hear slogans like "Treat yourself," "You do you," and "Live your truth," promoting the idea that personal gratification is the key to fulfillment. But is it true? The relentless pursuit of self-gratification often leads to shallow connections and fleeting approval. These are not the deep, meaningful relationships that nourish our need for connection—our need to love and be loved. Instead, they are transactional interactions with people who will move on as effortlessly as scrolling to the next post on their feed.

Divisiveness has become a defining feature of modern society, and it's deepening our crisis of disconnection. This is something I mentioned in the Introduction with polarizing groupthink, but it's a much broader societal problem. Instead of engaging in meaningful dialogue with those who hold different views, we ostracize and ignore them, retreating into echo chambers that reinforce our beliefs while alienating others. But make no mistake: We get what we give. This polarization erodes trust, weakens social bonds, and fuels isolation, as we lose the ability to see shared humanity beyond our disagreements.

The truth is, we are facing a growing epidemic of loneliness. In 2023, the US Surgeon General issued a special advisory, citing that before the pandemic half of Americans suffered from loneliness. Half! And that's before we sheltered in place, socially distanced, and wore masks. Elderly patients died alone in hospitals, while their loved ones said their final goodbyes through an iPad screen. Schools and workplaces went remote, isolating both children and adults in ways that we are still reckoning with today.

If we are to find our way back to fulfillment and well-being, we must reconnect—not just with others but with the deep, meaningful relationships that make us whole. One solution lies in the service of others. When we give to others—whether it's our time, our love, or our support—we find a deeper kind of validation: self-approval, self-esteem, and a profound sense of purpose that comes from sharing our gifts within a community built on mutual respect.

This shift in focus from self to others does not mean neglecting ourselves. Rather, it means understanding that the fulfillment we seek is in human connection. It means recognizing that our most important relationships, particularly with family, are the keys to unlocking our happiness. When we repair these bonds—when we build love and trust within our families—we release ourselves from the chains of resentment, fear, and loneliness. As Johann Hari, author of the book *Lost Connections*, beautifully stated, "Loneliness isn't the physical absence of people. It's a sense that we have nothing of value to share with anyone. To end loneliness, you need other people—plus something else.

You also need to feel you are sharing something with the other person or the group that is meaningful to both of you. You have to be in it together—and 'it' can be anything that you both think has meaning and value."

Spiritual Connection

Why am I here?
What is my purpose?
What will my life mean when I'm gone?

These questions are not trivial musings; they are the essence of our humanity. We are wired with a natural desire—a hunger—for understanding the bigger picture, for finding purpose, for knowing how we fit into the grand tapestry of existence. This longing is an inseparable part of the human experience, a persistent whisper in our hearts, urging us to seek deeper meaning and spiritual connection.

If we don't address these questions, life can feel unbearably hollow. If everything we do is reduced to a series of meaningless events, culminating in the inevitability of death, then the world becomes a dark, cruel, and purposeless place. This bleak perspective leaves us grappling with an existential anxiety—an unease about our own mortality and what lies beyond it.

It's worth it to spend some time searching for what makes life feel meaningful to you, what your purpose is. For me, it's faith in God. For many years, starting with college, I had drifted away, but as time went on, I began to feel that my soul needed to be fed—I could feel the hunger deep inside of me in that part that can't be seen, can't prove that it's a real thing, but I knew it was there. I knew I could partially feed that hunger with connection to other humans. But as philosopher Blaise Pascal once wrote, "There is a God-shaped hole in every human heart."

Connection to God was the only thing that would fill that space and fully satisfy me.

It's hardwired into us. Humanity radiated out across the globe, forming distinct cultures, civilizations, and histories that go back thousands of years—yet nearly every society arrived at the same basic truth: A higher power must be behind it all. In a world lacking physical proof of such a power, you would expect atheism to be the norm. Instead, across time and distance, people have consistently pointed to the sky, acknowledging that their higher power is up there. They may use different terms to describe it, but they converge on the same conclusion—that it exists. It's woven into who we are.

Science says that spiritual health is associated with less substance abuse; better coping with illness and adversity; less depression and anxiety; lower blood pressure; fewer strokes; less heart disease and Alzheimer's disease; and a longer life—basically, better emotional, physical, and cognitive health. On average, people who are spiritual are happier and more optimistic, and they have better self-esteem. Religious practice and spirituality are associated with lower markers of inflammation. There are many aspects of religion that activate the vagus nerve and pump the brakes on inflammation—prayer, singing, gratitude, and spiritual music. What we're talking about here is spiritual health, and I'm showing you that, much like emotional health, spiritual health affects your physiology and translates into physical health.

To be clear, I am not advocating for spirituality as a wellness hack. I am saying that there is a natural desire to satiate our hunger for a spiritual purpose, and when we do that, it contributes to our thriving—physically and emotionally. If you hear that whisper in your heart, you should listen to it. That's your soul talking to you.

Make no mistake. We all worship something. For many of us, it's our career and success, material things, political ideologies, some form of social activism, validation from a digital community, or some other form of self-identity. These aspects of life are like sugar for the soul.

They seem like a great idea, they taste good at the moment, but they don't actually satisfy you, and a few hours later you're even hungrier than when you started.

Usually the things that are most enriching about a spiritual practice include having a community of people with shared values and purpose; social support and acceptance; a sense of hope and optimism during times of adversity; moral guidance; altruism and acts of service that create connection; encouragement of forgiveness and emotional healing; and a framework for understanding mortality.

Spiritual purpose nourishes the soul in ways that defy explanation. It provides not just a sense of purpose but a profound feeling of belonging and a connection to something infinitely greater than ourselves. It becomes an anchor through the ups and downs, a constant reminder that we are wanted, valued, and endlessly loved. On the good days, we say thank you. And on the bad days, we draw comfort from God's boundless love, support, and peace—a reminder that we are never truly alone. Through faith in God, we recognize that our lives are not random—we are part of something eternal, placed here with intention and meaning.

A relationship with God offers an unwavering source of love, strength, and self-acceptance. In a world that can feel chaotic and isolating, God's presence remains steady. Perhaps you've noticed that being an adult isn't easy. There are triumphs and struggles, moments of joy and seasons of hardship. But God is always there. No matter what you face, you are a child of God, cherished beyond measure and loved unconditionally—yesterday, today, and for eternity.

The Healing Power of Awe

Have you ever been somewhere that sparks a sense of childlike wonder, and you start to take it all in—noticing the small details while simultaneously marveling at the grand scale? This is called having a sense of awe, and new research says that it activates our vagus nerve and reduces inflammation. In an eight-week study, they asked seniors seventy-five and older to take a fifteen-minute "awe" walk once per week. Basically, this meant pausing and taking time to appreciate the world around us. Just fifteen minutes and just once per week. By doing this, over time they had less distress and even less pain. But here's the interesting part: By expanding their attention to things other than themselves, they progressively became less focused on themselves and developed great feelings of social connection and compassion. The solution to societal narcissism is to see the world that exists beyond ourselves.

Healing Is Possible

My oldest daughter was born when I was thirty-three, and it was nothing short of life-changing. People tell you that something special happens when you have a child, but it's impossible to truly grasp until you experience it. For the first time, I felt the purpose I had been searching for. It was as if a missing piece of my soul clicked into place.

Becoming a parent gave me a deeper understanding of how my dad felt about me. I realized that he had loved me in the same way I now love my children—unconditionally, even through the imperfections and mistakes. I came to see that we, as humans, are fallible. But the love we share is real, vital, and worth fighting for. It's worth forgiving one another, so that our flaws don't become barriers to the connection and love that we so desperately need.

Parenthood also brought me closer to God. There's something truly miraculous about holding your child, feeling the weight of their tiny body, and realizing that their soul emerged from something far beyond science alone—it stands as evidence of something greater that transcends rational thought. The love I felt for my daughter gave me a glimpse of God's overwhelming love for me, gently unlocking and opening my heart to connect. For the first time, I truly felt worthy, purpose-driven, and capable of loving myself.

Around the time my daughter was born, I decided it was time to forgive my dad. After twelve years of silence, I called him. Reconnecting was transformative. It was a season of healing for both of us, as we made up for lost time. In September 2019, I traveled to Syracuse to see him. We spent the weekend revisiting our favorite things—watching a Syracuse football game, driving through the Adirondack Mountains, and even visiting the street where his grandparents, Polish immigrants, had lived.

That was the last time I saw my dad. He passed away unexpectedly in January 2020. I dedicated *Fiber Fueled* to him, and while I miss him dearly, I'm profoundly grateful that we were able to heal our relationship. My faith gives me peace, knowing he's in a better place and that we'll meet again someday. Our story isn't over.

Healing comes in many forms. We often think of it as the domain of medicine, but it's so much more than that. Food can be medicine, but so can connection. While isolation makes us weak, insecure, and fearful, connection gives us strength, confidence, and a sense of safety. Healing doesn't just happen in hospitals or through prescriptions—it happens in our relationships, in our communities, and in the quiet moments when we open our hearts.

What I witnessed in Dr. Drossman's clinic helped me see the profound connection between our mental, emotional, and spiritual health and our overall well-being. Life's traumas, disappointments, and unmet expectations can leave us feeling disconnected and unfulfilled. But healing begins when we face these wounds, reconnect with the people who matter most, and open ourselves to a higher power and purpose. This is not just about resolving past pain: It's about creating a foundation for a fulfilling future. It's time to take that step—to acknowledge your past, embrace your purpose, and find the healing that comes from love, connection, and faith.

Chapter 8 is backed by 179 references gathered through an extensive review of the scientific literature. You can browse the full citation list at www .theguthealthmd.com/plantpoweredplus.

PART III

FROM KNOWLEDGE TO ACTION, AND INSPIRATION TO TRANSFORMATION

CHAPTER 9

THE PLANT POWERED PLUS PROTOCOL

Welcome to the moment where knowledge turns into action and inspiration becomes transformation. Up to this point, we've explored the science of healing the microbiome, restoring the gut barrier, and empowering the immune system. We've uncovered the evidence that supports our approach. Now it's time to step into the driver's seat of your health journey. Welcome to the Plant Powered Plus Protocol, or as we'll call it moving forward, the P3 Protocol.

This chapter is your guide—a blueprint for reducing inflammation, optimizing gut-immune health, and building resilience. But more than that, it's your invitation to create a lifestyle deeply personal and powerful. This is not a one-size-fits-all mandate. It's not about obligations or following a rigid set of rules. It's about discovering what energizes you, what sparks your optimism, and what makes you excited to invest in your health. The only way to succeed with this protocol is to make it your own.

Before we dive in, let's talk about mindset. A growth mindset is the foundation of this protocol. It's the belief that your abilities and health are not fixed—that with effort, learning, and perseverance, you can improve. Challenges aren't obstacles to avoid; they're opportunities to grow, to gain new skills, and to build a stronger, healthier version of yourself.

Change isn't easy. The status quo is comfortable, even when it's killing you. You know it's time for change, but to actually make it happen is going to push you. That's why the P3 Protocol is organized around challenges. Each challenge is a chance to go beyond your comfort zone and unlock new skills while building momentum, confidence, and strength.

There will be victories, big and small, along the way. Celebrate them, but not too much—because every day, the sun rises again, and you'll have new opportunities. There will be setbacks, too. On those days, own the experience, learn from it, and move on. We don't want to let it stick. Negative energy doesn't serve you—it activates your sympathetic nervous system, creates inflammation, and zaps your energy. What does serve you is seeing every new day as a fresh start—a chance to keep building toward the healthiest version of yourself.

The closer you follow the protocol, the more you'll create synergies and raise the tide on your health, lifting everything up. But it's important to also be realistic. If you're feeling overwhelmed, scale back. Right-size the effort for you. Start small, grow steadily, and let your progress build over time.

This is a journey, not a race. The goal isn't to be perfect—it's to make progress. Look at where you started, where you are now, and where you're heading. Are you moving forward? That's what matters. Time is on your side, and this protocol is designed to flex with your needs. If you need more time in a phase, take it. The only timeline that matters is yours. My experience is that healing takes time, and it takes longer for some.

For some of you, the journey will be swift and linear. You'll dive in, take on all the challenges, and see results quickly. For others, the path will be more gradual. Both approaches are valid. Both lead to transformation and gut-immune health.

The P3 Protocol is your opportunity to take control of your health. It's your tool kit for reducing inflammation, restoring your gut, and empowering your immune system. The tools in this kit are evidence-based, so you can be confident that they will serve you well. The meal plan invites you to flourish by adding more—instead of restricting and depriving yourself. The challenges will help you take not only your physical health but also your emotional and spiritual health to a new level. The P3 Protocol is a celebration of your ability to grow, adapt, and thrive, and what lies ahead is a happier, healthier *you*.

So let's get started. Let's take action. Let's harness everything you've learned and turn it into something extraordinary. The path forward is clear, and it's yours to walk. Are you ready to take the challenge? Let's do this—one day, one step, and one sunrise at a time.

What's in the Protocol

The P3 Protocol is divided into three phases—**1: Baseline, 2: Growth,** and **3: Mastery**—each tailored to meet you where you are and guide you toward thriving health. Think of a phase as a period of personal development and substantial progress. You are working toward a specific goal that you establish at the beginning of each phase. A phase is not defined by a specific period of time. It's defined by your ability to accomplish your goals. The minimum required is at least a week per phase—three weeks total—to complete. For many of you it will take longer. Take as long as you need to achieve your goal.

In each phase, you will be presented with three important tools: your nutrition goals, a weekly meal plan, and a list of challenges to complete. There are shopping lists at my website—www.theguthealthmd.com. I encourage you to make this protocol your own. That means that you will review the full list of challenges at the beginning of each phase and determine which ones you are going to remove. There are also extra-credit challenges if you are rolling with positive momentum and you're so fired up that you're hungry for more. Or add them later.

Food is a part of all three phases of the P3 Protocol, and the recipes serve a specific purpose. As we discussed in Chapter 5, there are the four nutrition workhorses: fiber, polyphenols, healthy fats, and fermented foods. These are the four specific aspects of nutrition that are not only proven by science to nurture our gut microbiome and immune system, but also happen to be missing and wildly deficient for most people. Smart nutrition means addressing the parts of our diet that are not only missing but also most powerfully help us achieve our goals.

There are fifty-two recipes in this book, expertly developed by EA Stewart, a registered dietitian who specializes in nutrition for digestive health and autoimmune disease. I was thrilled to partner with EA—not only because of her professional expertise, but also because, like me, she has navigated her own health challenges. EA thrives with Sjögren's and, through dedicated research and trial and error, learned how to eat for her condition. This personal journey led her to develop an anti-inflammatory approach that she shares on her website, eastewart.com, empowering others to achieve better health.

Beyond her formal training, EA is a celebrated culinary expert known on social media as @TheSpicyRD. Her vibrant, healthful, science-backed recipes blend nutrition with flavor and have earned her numerous accolades. With her guidance, you can confidently embrace Plant Powered Plus nutrition, knowing that every recipe was created with care, creativity, and an unwavering commitment to your health goals.

Is the P3 Protocol Vegan, Vegetarian, Pescatarian, or Omnivorous?

The answer: Yes. I'm not a fan of diet labels; I'm a fan of dietary quality. Regardless of what dietary pattern you follow, I want to help you consume wholesome food that powers your gut microbes and health throughout your body. The P3 Protocol is here for *everyone* and isn't going to shoehorn you into a specific dietary pattern. Instead, I'm here to help you achieve your health goals by improving the quality of your diet and adding what's missing, not more of what you're already getting too much of.

The P3 Protocol starts 100 percent plant-based as a foundation because this creates the most flexibility for adaptation and individualization. You have the freedom to make it your own and to add the protein and optional ingredients that you prefer. Research has decisively shown that what matters is eating more of the good stuff. It's time to stop focusing on labels and just focus on eating quality whole foods.

In my experience, those who need the four workhorses the most are the ones who will struggle the most to add them. Why would that be? Well, it's no coincidence that the nutritional elements that impact our gut microbiome the most are also the ones that typically depend on the gut microbiome for digestion. Remember, fiber and resistant starch and most polyphenols are worthless until they come into contact with your gut microbes.

For this reason, the nutrition plan in the P3 Protocol is designed to start simple and progress to more complex. Imagine that you and I are both out on a boat on a beautiful day. Great music is playing and we're both wearing really cool shades, 'cause that's how we roll. There are two levers that I have my hand on to ease into our speed—digestibility and FODMAP content. Digestibility refers to how we cook and prepare the food to make it gentler and easier to digest. We start with smoothies and soups that are broken down and predigested in a way that makes it easier for our gut to get the nutrients we need with less work. As we push the throttle forward, we progress through other forms of cooking and preparation until, when we are at full throttle, we're including raw plant foods.

We approach FODMAPs in the same way. FODMAP is an acronym for fermentable oligosaccharides, disaccharides, monosaccharides, and polyols, which refer to the fermentable carbohydrates in some of our food. FODMAPs are poorly absorbed in the gut, leading to bloating, gas, and digestive distress in those with sensitive guts or conditions like IBS. Reducing FODMAP intake, which we call a low FODMAP diet, can reduce inflammation in the intestines and also improve gut symptoms, which is why it's a great place for us to start. However, many FODMAPs are prebiotic, making them essential for building gut health. When they are introduced strategically, tolerance to them builds as they feed and fuel our gut microbiome and it gets stronger and healthier. So the second lever in the P3 Protocol is FODMAP content, which starts low FODMAP and then progresses as we move forward.

You may be wondering about gluten. The P3 Protocol is designed to be low FODMAP—meaning high-FODMAP grains like wheat, barley, and rye are excluded—and as a result, all recipes are inherently gluten-free. There are some recipes that call for bread, and you get to choose what bread you use. I'd personally be opting for a nice organic sourdough. Two slices of fermented sourdough bread are low FODMAP, but not gluten-free. But you can keep the program 100 percent gluten-free if preferred.

Importantly, our goal is abundance and variety. As we've discussed throughout this book, your gut thrives on diversity. We know from the American Gut Project that those with the healthiest guts were the ones consuming at least thirty different plants per week. While most popular autoimmune protocols ask you to radically restrict your diet, I'm pushing you to go in a different direction—radical diversity. But that is built during the phases of the protocol as well.

Cooking for one, two, or your family? Plant Powered Plus includes recipes with varying servings, but you can easily adjust them to fit your needs. To scale a recipe up or down, multiply or divide the ingredient amounts accordingly. Always keep in mind that at each meal, you should eat until you're satisfied and according to your personal needs. If you need more food, consider adding a snack.

If you end up with leftovers, store them properly to maintain freshness, as specified in the "Pro Tips" section of the recipes. Most dishes keep well in airtight containers in the refrigerator for up to three or four days, while many soups and stews freeze beautifully for extended storage. For best results, label and date your leftovers, and when reheating, ensure they reach a safe internal temperature. With a little planning, you can enjoy delicious, homemade meals with minimal waste!

I know that many people out there are going to look at this book and the protocol and see a meal plan. But I want you to see that it's so much more. Your health and the health of your gut microbes are not exclusively defined by the foods that you eat. The opportunities for healing are vast and numerous, and we're intentionally taking advantage of *all* of that. I hope you'll be fired up to address all aspects of your physical, emotional, and spiritual health beyond your diet.

I said that most people do not have the four workhorses of Plant Powered Plus nutrition at the heart of their diet, but maybe that's not true for you. This is why the P3 Protocol is holistic. The missing piece *for you* may exist in the other aspects of health that you will be addressing. The beauty of it is that the protocol will help you find that and get it fixed, too.

Introducing the Three Phases of P3

The P3 Protocol is your road map to optimizing gut-immune health and reducing inflammation. It's designed to guide you through three transformative phases. Each phase builds on the previous one, empowering you to progress at your own pace while creating sustainable, long-term changes.

Phase 1: Baseline

Understand yourself, gently initiate the healing process, and establish sustainable habits

Your journey begins by first establishing the foundational elements that you need for thriving. I like to imagine that we're creating a thriving garden in your gut. In the first phase of gardening, we take our patch of dirt and prepare it. We remove the weeds and debris, till the soil, and plant the seeds. Although not required, we have the option to add some fertilizer to enhance it further. In this phase, you're not going to see much growing above the surface, but that's to be expected. The roots come before the shoots. We're creating the rich, supportive environment for a spectacular garden in the future.

The word I want you to think about in this phase is SUSTAINABLE. Whether it's diet or it's lifestyle, if it's not sustainable, then it's not going to work. We need to find what we can get to work in your life, because if it fits well, then it's here to stay, and you will receive the massive benefits that come from consistency.

In **Phase 1: Baseline**, nutrition will take somewhat of a back seat. Rather than adding too many new foods, we bring attention to the aspects of our diet that we're looking to pull back—sugar, refined carbs, salt, and fried food. At the same time, we're gently sneaking in more fiber, polyphenols, healthy fats, and fermented foods where there are opportunities. One way that we do this is by adding nutrient-dense smoothies and soups into your routine. Start each morning with a smoothie, add a gut-nourishing soup at lunch, and then enjoy a high polyphenol beverage as a nightcap.

This phase is an opportunity to spend your time and energy on establishing healthy habits. You'll have plenty of opportunity to grow in the kitchen, but first things first: Let's keep it simple and build our gut health with a few easy changes.

Phase 2: Growth
Balanced dietary expansion, addressing deficiencies, progress over perfection

In Phase 2, our gut garden is alive. You can see the juvenile sprouts rising up from the soil. At this point, they are weak and fragile, requiring careful attention to ensure that they thrive. Just as young plants need consistent watering, sunlight, and nutrients, your gut needs balanced nourishment, the resolution of deficiencies, and the cultivation of sustainable habits. This is the phase where growth happens—not through perfection, but through steady, deliberate progress. By enriching the soil of your microbiome with diverse plant foods, introducing healthy fats, and reinforcing your routines, you're fortifying these delicate sprouts into strong, resilient plants.

The word I want you to think about in this phase is CONSISTENCY. In Phase 1 we worked to identify sustainable diet and lifestyle choices. Hopefully you've identified many of those, and in this phase we want to focus on consistently doing them, locking them in. Your gut microbiome reacts and adapts to your choices—every one of them. When you create consistency around a choice, you nudge your microbiome along with you, and eventually that is how you create truly substantial change. Consistency is an essential concept for gut microbiome healing.

Let me be honest. **Phase 2: Growth** is probably the most challenging phase in the P3 Protocol. The reason for this is that we have the challenge of maintaining the habits that we installed in Baseline while adding new habits, taking them further, and simultaneously executing a dietary overhaul where we are cooking and eating new food.

Remember: The status quo is comfortable, even when it's killing you. Change is hard, even when it will heal you. We're making big changes in **Phase 2: Growth**. But your discipline will absolutely be rewarded. It's important to get yourself into that growth mindset, ready to take on the challenges knowing that at the top of the mountain not only does it get easier, but also there's something beautiful that's worth all of this effort and perseverance that you're investing. Also, there is no rush. Consistency plus time is the winning formula. Slow and steady wins over fast and fatigued.

Phase 3: Mastery
Gut-immune optimization, empowered gut health, building resilience

By this phase, your gut garden has transformed into a thriving ecosystem, lush with diversity and strength. The roots are deep, the plants are sturdy, and the garden is teeming with life. Not just plants, but you've attracted a few butterflies and hummingbirds, too! **Phase 3: Mastery** is about nurturing this ecosystem to its fullest potential—fine-tuning your habits, expanding your tolerance, and embracing advanced strategies to optimize your gut-immune connection. Like a seasoned gardener, you now understand your unique soil and environment, confidently cultivating resilience and balance. This is the stage where your garden not only thrives but becomes a source of lasting vitality, ready to withstand challenges and flourish through every season.

The word I want you to think about in this phase is OPTIMIZE. On many levels, life is about progress, staying committed to getting just 1 percent better. At no point should we stop in our pursuit of progress. You have heard me say that I want to address the most common and most important deficiencies—fiber, polyphenols, healthy fats, and fermented foods. But here's the thing . . . I'm not satisfied with you getting the minimum amount. That's like treating a D-minus the same as an A-plus, since they both constitute a pass. I want your health to be an A-plus. To get you there, we can't stop at D-minus; we must continue to optimize. That's what we are here to do in **Phase 3**, and that's what I want you to continue to do after. Keep progressing.

You will find that there's a far lighter burden of challenges in **Phase 3: Mastery**. That's because we're less focused on adding new changes. Instead, we are going to take what we've learned about ourselves from **Phase 1** and **Phase 2** and fine-tune it. Throughout this book we've discussed many different aspects of physical, emotional, and spiritual health. I want you to use **Phase 3: Mastery** as an opportunity to bring attention to whichever aspect of your health that you have been the least focused on thus far. It's most likely the thing that's hardest for you or that you're the most resistant to, and we can use this phase to invest energy in that specific area where we need it the most.

Ten Steps for Success with the P3 Protocol

Here are the key steps for using the P3 Protocol:

1 Review the Program and Personalize It

Spend some time reviewing and thoughtfully considering this program. The goal is to make it your own. Identify which challenges align with your needs and lifestyle, and remove those that don't. This way, you focus on what works best for you.

Reasons to remove challenges or recipes may include:

- **Health considerations:** A condition that prevents you from doing it. Discuss with your doctor.

- **Schedule conflicts:** Incompatibility with your routine. Do the best you can to resolve these.

- **Accessibility:** Lack of access or availability. Consider similar alternatives.

- **Cost:** Financial constraints. Explore more affordable or free alternatives.

- **Cultural or religious reasons:** I respect that. Honor your values and traditions and find a way to do what works for you.

If anything requires consultation with your health care provider, make notes so you're prepared for that discussion. And remember, you can always add back the challenges that you've removed later.

2 Complete Pre-Protocol Work

Before diving in, prepare by:

- **Familiarizing yourself with Chapters 1–8 of this book.**

- **Meeting with your health care provider** to discuss specific aspects of your health or perform necessary testing.

- **Reviewing page 376 of the Appendix,** where you'll find tips I encourage but that aren't formally in the P3 Protocol. You can implement these now or work on them later.

3 Plan Before Starting Each Phase

Before starting a new phase:

- **Review the challenges and recipes** again and remove any that won't work for you. Pay attention to the serving sizes and determine how much of each recipe (and the ingredients) you'll need.

- **Determine your pace:** Decide if you'll move quickly and tackle multiple challenges or ease in gradually.

- **Define success:** Set a specific, measurable goal to track your progress. Begin monitoring before the phase starts.

4 Create a Weekly Checklist

Once you have reviewed the challenges and pruned the ones that you won't be doing, create a checklist for the week that will allow you to check off each challenge for each of the seven days. The easiest way to do this is to write the list of challenges on the left side of a piece of paper and then add seven checkboxes, one for each day of the week, to the right of each. Obviously, you could use your computer to help facilitate this if you prefer, or you can go full-scale journal style with a pencil and keep it old school. I'll have resources available to you on my website—www.theguthealthmd.com/plantpoweredplus—if desired. Your job is to take the P3 Protocol from this book and transfer it into a format that results in action.

5 Monitor How You Feel

What matters is how you feel—your energy levels, digestive comfort, physical ease, mood, and sleep. To know if you're truly improving, you need to track these changes. We'll dive into the details shortly, but for now, just remember that documenting how you feel each day is key to understanding your progress. If you don't track these changes, you won't know if you're truly improving—so let's make it part of the plan.

6 Don't Bite Off More Than You Can Chew

There are extra-credit challenges, and it's tempting to tackle them all at once—especially on Day 1. But that can be overwhelming. Don't feel obligated to do *all* of them. Sustainability is a nonnegotiable, so I want you to start with what you actually are willing and able to do. You can always add more later, including the extra-credit challenges.

7 Commit to Growth and Stay Flexible

Focus on progress over perfection. Life will throw curveballs, and that's okay. Don't ever feel shame or feel defeated. Don't even let those thoughts enter your mind. Do your best. Sometimes it's one step backward before two steps forward. Embrace that. Be kind to yourself, adapt when needed, and celebrate what you're doing right. Discipline matters—hang in there; your efforts will be rewarded.

8 Aim for Clear and Substantial Progress

Each phase lasts as long as it takes to achieve clear, substantial progress. You are working toward a specific goal that you establish at the beginning of each phase. Track your progress toward your goal. When you've introduced the daily challenges for a phase and maintained improvement for three consecutive days, you're ready to move forward.

9 Build Upon Each Phase

The P3 Protocol is cumulative. You're not starting over with each phase—you're growing. Think of it like a pyramid, with every challenge being a brick. In the beginning, you're laying the broad, strong foundation. As you progress, the pyramid is growing taller and the last bricks are much more focused and tactical. Each new phase builds on the last, adding skills and tools while maintaining previous progress.

10 Repeat the Process

When you're ready for the next phase, return to Step 3 and repeat. You're steadily cultivating resilience, thriving health, and an empowered gut-immune system.

Measuring Your Progress: Your N of 1 Study

The P3 Protocol is not a one-size-fits-all approach. It's a personal journey—your "N of 1" study. In research, the term *N* refers to the number of participants in a study, and larger studies with more participants provide better insight into what we can expect in a population of people. But let's be honest: What happens with ten thousand other people isn't what really matters when it comes to your health. What matters is how this protocol impacts *you*.

An "N of 1" study is an experiment of one—you. You become the scientist of your own health, observing and recording your experiences and outcomes. The beauty of this approach is its focus on individuality: your unique body, challenges, and progress. It helps you find what works specifically for you.

At the heart of this process is having a specific health goal that you're tracking and trying to improve. Some of you may be tempted to use microbiome testing, blood work, or a health measure from your wearable device as your health goal, but I'm putting my foot down: That's not what we're going to do. I want you to focus on how you feel. If we met in a clinic, I'd walk into the room and sit down at your eye level and ask you, "How are you feeling?"

Yes, I would review your microbiome results and blood work and would find your HRV (heart rate variability) very interesting. I'd absolutely look at those things because they provide insights. But I don't treat numbers, I treat people, and the most accurate and telling reflection of a person's health is how that person feels. That means that for your specific health goal, I want you to choose from this list:

- Energy levels (physical vitality)
- Digestive comfort
- Menopause or menstrual comfort
- Physical comfort (such as joint comfort)
- Mood and emotional stability
- Mental clarity
- Hunger control and cravings
- Physical performance (exercise)

You need to choose where you have the most to gain, but if you're unsure, then let me propose that you use energy levels. Energy is an excellent barometer of health. We all know how it feels to be energized versus fatigued. Energy levels matter to everyone, and they naturally rise when we're thriving and fall when we're unwell.

Research has shown that inflammation plays a significant role in this connection. When inflammation rises, energy levels drop. This was clearly shown in a study where healthy humans were injected with lipopolysaccharide (LPS), and inflammation levels and fatigue rose in parallel. Growing evidence suggests that neuroinflammation, meaning inflammation of the brain, manifests with fatigue. It's no coincidence that chronic inflammatory conditions like autoimmune disease are strongly associated with fatigue, to the point that 98 percent report its presence. But even in a healthy population, up to 45 percent report persistent fatigue. As we've learned in this book and I've shown you in the table on page 371, we are facing an epidemic of chronic inflammation. It's no surprise that so many of us have low energy levels.

That said, energy levels aren't solely tied to inflammation. For instance, if you have diabetes or irregular blood sugar, these can also influence your energy. You'd also feel low energy if you are in a calorie deficit, or if you are dehydrated or have nutrient deficiencies. Choose energy as your barometer if it aligns with your health journey, but know that other measures—like mood or digestive comfort—can be equally valid.

It's important to create a simple and effective system to monitor your progress that works for you. I love the idea of a journal that allows you to reflect on how you're doing. Start with your primary metric that you selected from the list above—energy, mood, digestive comfort, etc. Record it daily on a 0–10 scale, ideally at the same time of day. You can keep it easy and use a calendar or sheet of paper to record your score daily. You also can get as crazy as you want and use a spreadsheet with additional data such as HRV, resting heart rate (RHR), or even blood work results. Feel free to track more than one measure if that's important to you, but you are required to select only the one primary metric that will define your journey. If you'd prefer a ready-made template, head over to **www.theguthealthmd.com/plantpoweredplus**, where you can download worksheets, join my email community, and get ongoing tips and support to keep you on track.

Clear and substantial progress is defined by *your* satisfaction with the result. To ensure your baseline reflects a true area of improvement, your starting score should fall between 2 and 7. If you're already a 9 at baseline, then you need to choose a different metric or stop inflating your score. At the start of each phase, set a clear goal. For example, aim for your primary metric to improve by at least two points from baseline. A phase is considered complete when you have fulfilled the essentials challenges *and* achieved clear and substantial progress with your health goal.

Remember: This is your journey. Monitor it, refine it, and celebrate it. The P3 Protocol is about growth, and with each phase, you're building a healthier, more resilient you. Trust the process, and let your health story unfold one step at a time.

Complementing Your Journey with Wearable Technology

If you enjoy collecting data, two metrics from wearable devices that I trust are heart rate variability (HRV) and resting heart rate (RHR). HRV is a measure of the variability between heartbeats, reflecting the balance between your sympathetic (stress) and parasympathetic (rest and digest) nervous systems. When your parasympathetic is more active, there's more variability between beats, which leads to higher HRV. It's important to understand that your HRV is not like blood work, where there are standard measures that define health versus disease. Instead, HRV is meant to be seen as relative, meaning that you should interpret against your own measures, not against other people's. In general, higher HRV indicates better adaptability and resilience. Meanwhile, your resting heart rate is a measure of how many times your heart beats per minute while at rest. Lower RHR generally reflects better cardiovascular fitness and a more relaxed nervous system. You'll generally find that low RHR correlates with high HRV. These secondary measures are helpful and worthy of tracking, but they should never overshadow your primary focus on how you feel.

What to Do If It's Not Going Well

Come back to this page when you need it. Healing is a journey, not a linear path, and it's completely normal to encounter challenges along the way, especially if you're starting with a significantly damaged gut. I believe wholeheartedly that your gut can and will heal when properly supported. But this process requires time, patience, and consistency. Sometimes it feels slow—or even nonexistent—but don't lose sight of the long game: Healing takes time, and you're laying the groundwork for a better, healthier future.

For those with damaged gut health, food intolerances can be a significant hurdle. You might find certain foods difficult to tolerate, and that's okay. The first thing to do is ask yourself whether there's a medical issue that could be holding you back, such as chronic constipation, flaring inflammatory bowel disease, or unstable blood sugar control. It's important to address those issues directly with your health care provider. While the P3 Protocol is designed to support healing, it's not meant to replace medical therapy. Sometimes addressing these medical concerns is what unlocks the ability to tolerate more foods and implement the lifestyle changes needed for deeper healing. Short-term medical support can set the stage for long-term success by helping you tolerate more foods and deeper lifestyle changes.

You should also be aware of potential triggers. These can come in many forms—certain foods, environmental factors, stress, or even lifestyle habits that may seem harmless at first. Triggers are highly individual, and what affects one person may not bother another, which is why paying close attention to your body's signals is so important. The key is to approach this process with curiosity and a willingness to experiment. If you suspect something might be triggering your symptoms, try removing it temporarily and observing how your body responds. This isn't about creating unnecessary restrictions but rather about finding the balance that allows your body to thrive.

For many people, introducing more fiber or FODMAP-rich foods is difficult. It's not particularly surprising, because these are the foods that we *need* our microbiome to help us with, and their abilities may be hindered when the gut is damaged. Similarly, a damaged gut barrier may make high-histamine foods—fermented foods, fish and shellfish, spinach, tomatoes, and avocados—more difficult to handle. Histamine intolerance is not a topic of focus in this book, but it was covered heavily in *The Fiber Fueled Cookbook*. If high fiber, FODMAPs, or histamine foods are difficult for you, start low and go slow—and feel free to slow down even more whenever you need to. I'm providing a list of low FODMAP foods in the Appendix (page 373) that you can reference if you need it. Remember, what matters is success, not how quickly you get there. But if resolving these issues on your own isn't working, consider partnering with a registered dietitian who can guide you in a more tailored way.

It may be that part of the P3 Protocol itself is not the right match for you at a certain moment. You have to make the program your own from the start. Perhaps the time-restricted eating interval feels too long, or maybe you're feeling stuck with the emotional or spiritual aspects of the program. This is where reflection becomes essential. Take a step back and ask yourself if there's something specific in the protocol that feels like it's holding you back. If so, you have two options: Adapt it to better fit your needs, or remove it temporarily. Don't feel like you've failed if you need to modify the plan—it's designed to be flexible. Sometimes doing less and doing it well is the best way forward, especially if the alternative is feeling overwhelmed by doing too much. Keep moving forward, even if the steps feel small. Trust the process, trust your body, and remember that healing is happening, even when it feels slow.

Laboratory Monitoring

Laboratory monitoring can be a valuable tool for tracking your health progress and assessing how your body responds to the P3 Protocol, but it's important to emphasize that this is not a requirement for success. I've already made my argument for why I want you to focus on how you feel. However, for those who enjoy a more data-driven approach, blood work can provide an additional layer of insight into your gut and immune health. And absolutely, as a medical doctor, I would incorporate these test results into my understanding of what's happening with you. But I would caution you that laboratory interpretation can be highly complex and require expertise to understand the complete context, and for this reason I would never want you to test and interpret independently unless you yourself are a qualified health care professional. It is for this reason that I am not providing target numbers for each of these, because context is required for that and it should be personalized.

The list of tests provided here serves as a foundational starting point that's meant to be widely applicable, offering broad insights into inflammation, nutrient status, and gut-related health markers. If you have a specific health condition, such as an autoimmune disease, you may need to expand this list to include more specialized tests, such as autoantibodies or other markers that relate directly to your condition. For example, if you have symptoms with gluten-containing foods, you absolutely should pursue testing for celiac disease as described in Chapter 5. You may not need every one of these tests as well, or you may check them at baseline and find that they are already normal and ongoing monitoring may not be necessary. With all of these questions, it is best to work with your health care provider.

I recommend checking these markers at baseline to establish a clear starting point and then repeating them every three to six months. This allows you and your health care provider to assess trends, make adjustments to your protocol, and ensure that your progress aligns with your health goals. Even if you complete a phase or more than one phase of the protocol, you want to provide enough time for laboratory results to catch up and for the updated results to be meaningful.

TEST NAME	WHAT IT MEASURES	RELATION TO GUT HEALTH AND INFLAMMATION
White blood cells (part of Complete Blood Count)	White blood cells are part of the immune system	High levels indicate infection, inflammation, or stress. Very low levels can indicate infections, autoimmune diseases, or bone marrow issues.
Hemoglobin (part of Complete Blood Count)	The protein in red blood cells that carries oxygen	Low indicates anemia, while high may indicate dehydration.
Platelets (part of Complete Blood Count)	Cells involved in blood clotting	High levels can be caused by inflammation.
C-reactive Protein (CRP)	A marker of systemic inflammation	Elevated levels indicate acute or chronic inflammation in the body.
Erythrocyte Sedimentation Rate (ESR)	The rate at which red blood cells settle in a test tube	Another marker of total body inflammation that is used alongside CRP for a fuller picture of inflammation.
LPS-Binding Protein (LBP)	A protein produced by the liver in response to the presence of LPS	High levels are associated with systemic inflammation and gut barrier compromise.
Vitamin D (25-hydroxyvitamin D)	Vitamin D levels in the blood	Critical for gut barrier function, immune regulation, and reducing inflammation.
Omega-3 Index	Percentage of EPA and DHA in red blood cell membranes	Reflects anti-inflammatory omega-3 status, which is important for gut and immune health.
Fasting Comprehensive Metabolic Panel (CMP)	Electrolytes, kidney function, liver enzymes, and blood sugar	Offers insight into overall metabolic health, hydration, and organ function.
Fasting Insulin	Insulin levels before food	When combined with fasting blood sugar, allows determination of HOMA-IR, a measure of insulin resistance.
Hemoglobin A1c (HbA1c)	Provides a longer-term view of blood sugar control	Long-term blood sugar control is closely linked to inflammation and gut health.

TEST NAME	WHAT IT MEASURES	RELATION TO GUT HEALTH AND INFLAMMATION
Prealbumin	A measure of nutritional status	Decreased during inflammation and can provide nutritional insight for those with poor gut health, such as inflammatory bowel disease.
Fasting Lipid Panel (Cholesterol, HDL, LDL, triglycerides)	Measures of blood lipids	Helps evaluate cardiovascular health and inflammation linked to metabolic function.
Apolipoprotein B (ApoB)	A protein that carries the unhealthy cholesterol	A better predictor of cardiovascular risk than LDL cholesterol, once again linked to metabolic health.
Ferritin	Iron storage levels	Low levels can suggest iron deficiency; high levels may indicate inflammation or iron overload.
Zinc	A trace mineral essential for immune function and wound healing	Maintains gut barrier integrity and is anti-inflammatory.
Magnesium	A mineral involved in more than three hundred enzymatic reactions	Regulates gut motility, reduces gut inflammation, supports gut microbial balance and barrier function.
Vitamin B_{12}	A water-soluble vitamin	Deficiency is common and it is crucial for energy metabolism..
Homocysteine	Amino acid level	Elevated levels can be a marker of inflammation and poor methylation.
Thyroid Panel (TSH, Free T4)	Thyroid function	Thyroid dysfunction can impact gut motility and inflammation, and thyroid autoimmunity can overlap with gut issues.
Fecal Calprotectin	Protein in stool linked to inflammation	Helps assess gut inflammation, particularly in inflammatory bowel disease.
Fecal Lactoferrin	A protein released by neutrophils during inflammation	Elevated when there is significant inflammation in the intestines.
Fecal Alpha-1 Antitrypsin	A protein produced in the liver that is detected in stool when there is intestinal inflammation or a compromised gut barrier	Elevated levels may indicate ongoing gut damage in the context of inflammatory bowel disease or celiac disease.
Stool Microbiome Analysis	Microbial diversity and composition	Optional but insightful for gut health.

A Heartfelt Message from Dr. B

Before you embark on your journey and having spent some time now with you, I want to take a moment to share a few thoughts with you about this book. It took me not just months but years to write. I threw myself with focus and vigor into a simple question: What are the steps that a person can take to heal their gut microbiome and, as a result, empower a stronger immune system? My focus has been and will always be on the individual people who I am trying to help. Forget selling books and social media followers and all of the pageantry for a moment. At my core, my childhood dream was to be a doctor and help people. It's the fabric of my soul. As my career has evolved, I've found new ways to fulfill this goal, but my heart and focus remain on that individual who needs healing. This is my way of saying that I wrote this book for you. You were meant to find it, read it, and have it do something meaningful for you. Where you are in this moment, and what you're about to do, is what motivated and inspired me through the grueling effort that I put into this book. The fact that you have given me your time and attention is the greatest honor for me. This book is more than just a guide; it's a partnership between us, built on trust and a shared goal of transforming your health. Now it's time to make it happen. There will be challenges along the way, but I believe in your ability to rise above them, step by step, day by day. Just know that I am with you in spirit, cheering you on through every twist and turn. Let's embark on this journey together, with hope, determination, and the belief that healing is possible.

Chapter 9 is backed by 11 references gathered through an extensive review of the scientific literature. You can browse the full citation list at www .theguthealthmd.com/plantpoweredplus.

PHASE 1: BASELINE

Goals: Understand yourself, gently initiate the healing process, and establish sustainable habits

In **Phase 1: Baseline**, we are creating the ideal environment for your gut and immune systems to flourish. We are guided by the mantra "start low and go slow." "Start low" in this phase means adding in a few low FODMAP foods. It also means preparing foods in a way that makes them easier on our gut, with smoothies and soups.

The smoothies, soups, and beverages in this phase aren't intended to be your only meals. But we are slowly shifting you to more plants, allowing your gut to get exposed to and adapted to them.

As you prepare for this phase, be aware that you will be using your blender daily, sometimes a few times daily. Make sure that you have a blender that you're happy with before you get started. It makes sense to batch cook the soup recipes, and you can do this ahead if you prefer.

During this phase we also are going to build out our morning and evening routines and other lifestyle elements that will form the foundation for our health. Throughout this process, maintain your gaze on the importance of consistency and connection. Take it slowly, be patient, and trust the process.

Recipes for **Phase 1: Baseline** include three smoothies, three soups, and four drinks. To keep you organized and on top of things, here I provide you with clarity and structure for a few specifics: a list of Phase 1 foods to prioritize or limit, an optional meal plan, and a daily checklist for lifestyle measures. Please note that the meal plan and daily checklist can and should be adjusted to your needs and preferences and how many people you are cooking for.

Phase 1 Nutrition Guidelines

Prioritize	10+ different plants per week
	Low FODMAP plant-based foods: fruits, vegetables, whole grains, seeds, nuts, legumes (see page 373 for list)
	Add extra greens to your smoothies and soups
	Add extra chia seeds, flaxseeds, hempseeds, and basil seeds to smoothies
	Make sure to get varied colors among your plant foods, for more polyphenol variety
	Polyphenol drinks: green and black tea, herbal tea, coffee, kombucha
	Spices are your polyphenol-rich friends
	When you need a snack, focus on fruit and nuts or a smoothie
	When you need a sweet treat, opt for dark chocolate or berries
	Fermented plant-based foods
Allowed	Low FODMAP protein powder (plain brown rice protein or a certified low FODMAP protein) in smoothies to make it a meal replacement and fulfill protein needs
	Extra-virgin olive oil
	If consuming animal products, prioritize fish and shellfish, fermented dairy, and eggs
	Sourdough bread (if tolerating gluten)
	High FODMAP plant-based foods, if tolerated (see page 374 for list)
	Raw vegetables, if tolerated
Off-Limits	Added sugar or artificial sweeteners except fermented drinks (stevia and monk fruit are okay)
	Gluten and flour except sourdough
	Salty snacks
	Fried foods
	Sugary desserts or candy
	Processed meats
	Fast food

Phase 1 Weekly Meal Plan

DAY 1		
FAST BREAKING SMOOTHIE	**LUNCHTIME SOUP**	**EVENING BEVERAGE**
Golden Green Kickstart Smoothie	P3 Biome Broth	Citrus-Spiced Golden Milk

DAY 2		
FAST BREAKING SMOOTHIE	**LUNCHTIME SOUP**	**EVENING BEVERAGE**
Citrus Berry Belly Bliss Smoothie	Sun-Kissed Curry Carrot Soup	Ginger Green Refresher

DAY 3		
FAST BREAKING SMOOTHIE	**LUNCHTIME SOUP**	**EVENING BEVERAGE**
Oatmeal Cookie Dough Smoothie	Sun-Kissed Curry Carrot Soup	Tropic Mint Kiwi Cooler

DAY 4		
FAST BREAKING SMOOTHIE	**LUNCHTIME SOUP**	**EVENING BEVERAGE**
Golden Green Kickstart Smoothie	P3 Biome Broth	The Blue Zen Elixir

DAY 5		
FAST BREAKING SMOOTHIE	**LUNCHTIME SOUP**	**EVENING BEVERAGE**
Citrus Berry Belly Bliss Smoothie	Creamy Cannellini and Parsnip Soup	Ginger Green Refresher

DAY 6		
FAST BREAKING SMOOTHIE	**LUNCHTIME SOUP**	**EVENING BEVERAGE**
Oatmeal Cookie Dough Smoothie	P3 Biome Broth	The Blue Zen Elixir

DAY 7		
FAST BREAKING SMOOTHIE	**LUNCHTIME SOUP**	**EVENING BEVERAGE**
Golden Green Kickstart Smoothie	Creamy Cannellini and Parsnip Soup	Tropic Mint Kiwi Cooler

WEEK 1 PLANT TOTAL: 38 UNIQUE PLANTS

NOTES ON PHASE 1 MEAL PLAN:

- If you'd like a shopping list for Phase 1, head to my website—www
  .theguthealthmd.com/plantpoweredplus.

- Each smoothie is a single serving and best prepared and consumed fresh. You are encouraged to break your fast with a smoothie each day.

- If you choose to follow the meal plan exactly and use P3 Biome Broth instead of water or store-bought broth in all the Phase 1 soup recipes, you'll need 16 cups of broth total. One batch of P3 Biome Broth makes about 10 cups, so double the recipe and refrigerate or freeze the leftovers for later.

- Each of the three soups can be batch prepared and stored in the fridge for up to 4 days, with leftovers frozen for up to 6 months.

- The Ginger Green Refresher (Days 2 and 5) can be made fresh each time or prepared in a slightly bigger batch on Day 2 and refrigerated up to 4 days. Shake well before serving.

- The Blue Zen Elixir yields about 4 servings per batch and can be stored for up to 1 week in the fridge. You need only 2 servings across the week, but you are encouraged to drink more or to carry forward the leftover into the next week.

Phase 1 Daily Checklist

MORNING
- ○ 2 glasses water
- ○ Morning supplements at <u>scheduled</u> time
  - Low FODMAP prebiotic supplement (start low, go slow) (see cheat sheet, page 173)
  - Vitamin D (see cheat sheet, page 179)

- ◌ Omega-3 (see cheat sheet, page 181)
- ◌ Turmeric supplement (start 500 milligrams and increase to 1,000 milligrams) (see cheat sheet, page 189)
- ○ 30 minutes sunlight
- ○ 3–5 minutes breathwork training

EVENING
- ○ No caffeine or carbonated drinks
- ○ No solid food after 8:00 p.m.
- ○ Minimize light exposure: dim lighting, blue light filters, digital detox
- ○ Evening supplements at <u>scheduled</u> time
  - ◌ Melatonin supplement: low and slow, 0.5–3 milligrams 60–90 minutes before bed (see cheat sheet, page 182)
  - ◌ Zinc supplement (see cheat sheet, page 185)
  - ◌ Magnesium supplement (see cheat sheet, page 184)
- ○ 3–5 minutes breathwork
- ○ Consistent bedtime
- ○ 7–8 hours in bed

LIFESTYLE
- ○ No alcohol, tobacco, or marijuana
- ○ Turn off phone at mealtimes
- ○ 30 minutes exercise (brisk walk, cardio, resistance training)

PHASE 1 HOMEWORK
(DO ONCE EACH PHASE)
- ○ Schedule a phone call or coffee to connect with a friend or loved one.
- ○ Reflect on how stress, emotions, and past experiences affect your physical health. Is there an open wound from your past

that needs to be addressed? Is there something in your present that's holding you back? If so, discuss with a loved one or health professional to create a plan to address it.

○ Reflect on your relationships with others. Who are the people who lift you up and make you feel whole?

○ Reflect on what gives your life meaning. What is your purpose? How spiritually fulfilled are you?

○ Take a weekly 15-minute "awe walk" to appreciate nature and spark a sense of wonder.

EXTRA CREDIT

○ Add 1 new fermented food.

○ Extra omega-3-rich foods

○ Extra leafy greens

○ 3 days in a row home-cooked food

○ Try sprouts.

○ Add a squeeze of citrus or splash of apple cider vinegar to water or other beverages.

○ Explore calming evening beverages: chamomile tea, valerian root tea, or tart cherry juice.

○ Deep breathing exercises around mealtimes

○ Experiment with techniques to stimulate the vagus nerve as provided on page 207 (Chapter 8).

○ Reduce screen time.

When Are You Done with Phase 1?

At a minimum, Phase 1 should last one week. Hopefully, as I recommended on page 245, you have identified a primary health goal and have been tracking your progress by scoring how you feel, on a scale from 0 to 10 on a daily basis. Our focus in Phase 1 is to experience clear and substantial progress toward that goal. You may not have fulfilled that health goal completely, but you want to be feeling better than when you started. If after one week you're not there yet, I'd encourage you to continue in Phase 1. You can repeat the meal plan or you can replace the daily smoothie, soup, and beverage provided the replacement is also low FODMAP. You will find such recipes in *The Fiber Fueled Cookbook*, Chapter 4.

PHASE 2: GROWTH

Goals: Balanced dietary expansion, addressing deficiencies, progress over perfection

In **Phase 2: Growth**, we transition from laying the foundation to actively nurturing and strengthening the progress we've made. This phase is about progress over perfection—embracing the challenges and opportunities for growth. You'll build from where you were in Phase 1. This means that you should take what worked for you in Phase 1 and keep at it! We don't want to stop using the lifestyle and nutrition tweaks that are helping us.

Now let's go one further. In Phase 2 you'll find what you need to level up your health—updated nutrition guidelines, a new meal plan for the week, a fresh daily checklist, and new extra-credit challenges. As you've done already, make sure that you are tailoring your approach to fit your unique needs.

I want you to take notice of your progress. Yes, progress is measured by how you're coming along with your health goal. We absolutely want to see that. But just as importantly, progress is measured by your perseverance and ability to set a goal and follow through on it. This helps you foster greater confidence in your ability to persevere, which is what you need to heal and thrive. The goal is not only to grow in Phase 2 but also to feel encouraged by your ability to change and adapt and progress, one step at a time.

In Phase 2, your diet will be fully Plant Powered. This means that I will be providing you with breakfast, lunch, and dinner recipes every day. You will have snack and sweet options. The recipes for Phase 2 include six breakfasts, seven entrées, two soups, and four snacks and sweets. I would like for you to start each morning with a smoothie. Breakfast is optional; it's your choice whether or not to include it. Add the snacks and desserts as desired, particularly if you're hungry between lunch and dinner. Add the polyphenol-rich beverages from Phase 1 as desired.

Phase 2 Nutrition Guidelines

Prioritize	20+ different plants per week *UPDATED*
	80+ percent whole foods (20 percent or less ultra-processed foods) *NEW*
	Resistant starches—cooked and cooled potatoes or sweet potatoes, legumes, whole grains *NEW*
	Add more healthy fats (EVOO, avocado, nuts, fish/shellfish) *NEW*
	Fermented foods daily *NEW*
	Low FODMAP plant-based foods: fruits, vegetables, whole grains, seeds, nuts, legumes (see page 373 for list)
	Make sure to get varied colors among your plant foods, for more polyphenol variety
Allowed	Low FODMAP protein powder (plain brown rice protein or a certified low FODMAP protein) in smoothies if skipping breakfast
	Extra-virgin olive oil
	If consuming animal products, prioritize fish and shellfish, fermented dairy, and eggs
	Sourdough bread (if tolerating gluten)
	High FODMAP plant-based foods, if tolerated (see page 374 for list)
	Raw vegetables, if tolerated

Off-Limits	Added sugar or artificial sweeteners except fermented drinks (stevia and monk fruit are okay)
	Gluten and flour except sourdough
	Salty snacks
	Fried foods
	Sugary desserts or candy
	Processed meats
	Fast food

Phase 2 Weekly Meal Plan

DAY 1

BREAKFAST	LUNCH	DINNER
Wild Blueberry Chia Crisp with Yogurt	Citrus-Kissed Cannellini Stew	Herby Chickpea Quinoa Salad

DAY 2

BREAKFAST	LUNCH	DINNER
Orange and Spice Overnight Oats	Miso-Licious Vegetable Pasta	Sweet Potato Lentil Curry

DAY 3

BREAKFAST	LUNCH	DINNER
Tropical Chia Pudding	Herby Chickpea Quinoa Salad (Day 1 leftovers)	Creamy Miso-Peanut Noodle Bowl

DAY 4

BREAKFAST	LUNCH	DINNER
Kimchi Tofu Scramble Breakfast Tacos	Sweet Potato Lentil Curry (Day 2 leftovers)	Garden Green Spud Salad

DAY 5

BREAKFAST	LUNCH	DINNER
Cinnamon Crunch Buckwheat Granola	Rosemary Minestrone Soup	Wild Rice Power Bowl

DAY 6		
BREAKFAST	**LUNCH**	**DINNER**
Wild Blueberry Smoothie Bowl	Garden Green Spud Salad (Day 4 leftovers)	Easy Stir-Fried Veggie and Edamame Rice

DAY 7		
BREAKFAST	**LUNCH**	**DINNER**
Orange and Spice Overnight Oats	Wild Rice Power Bowl (Day 5 leftovers)	Rosemary Minestrone Soup

Phase 2 Optional Recipes

SMOOTHIES	SNACKS AND SWEETS	BEVERAGES	PROTEIN ADD-ONS
Start your morning with a smoothie.	Listen to your hunger cues between lunch and dinner.	Add polyphenol-rich beverages throughout the day.	Flexible proteins to add as desired to your meals.
Golden Green Kickstart Smoothie (page 281)	Edamame Guacamole (page 319)	Ginger Green Refresher (page 278)	Crispy Baked Tofu (page 362)
Citrus Berry Belly Bliss Smoothie (page 282)	Citrus and Herb Toasted Nut Mix (page 320)	Citrus-Spiced Golden Milk (page 279)	The *Best* Tempeh (page 363)
	5-Ingredient Energy Bites (page 321)	The Blue Zen Elixir (page 280)	Soft/Medium/Hard–Boiled Eggs (page 365)
	Chocolate Raspberry Chia Parfait (page 322)	Tropic Mint Kiwi Cooler (page 283)	Easy Pan-Seared Salmon (page 366)
	Fruits	Green and black tea	Stovetop Shrimp (page 367)
	Nuts	Herbal tea	
	Smoothie	Coffee	
	Berries	Kombucha	
	Dark chocolate		

WEEK 2 PLANT TOTAL: 66 UNIQUE PLANTS

NOTES ON PHASE 2 MEAL PLAN:

- If you'd like a shopping list for Phase 2, head to my website—www .theguthealthmd.com/plantpoweredplus.

- Each smoothie is a single serving and best prepared and consumed fresh. You are encouraged to break your fast with a smoothie each day.

- If you plan to use your P3 Biome Broth in all of these recipes, you will need around 18 cups of broth. That would require you to make two batches of broth, which have 10 cups each.
  » Citrus-Kissed Cannellini Stew (Day 1 Lunch)—6 cups total
  » Sweet Potato Lentil Curry (Day 2 Dinner)—4–6 cups total
  » Rosemary Minestrone Soup (Days 5 Lunch + 7 Dinner)— 6 cups per batch

- To streamline your efforts, we'll use leftovers from the five dinner recipes below to create other dinners a couple of days later. For each of these meals, you will want to make sure you are preparing extra so that you'll have enough to use again.
  » Herby Chickpea Quinoa Salad—Day 1 Dinner
  » Sweet Potato Lentil Curry—Day 2 Dinner
  » Garden Green Spud Salad—Day 4 Dinner
  » Rosemary Minestrone Soup—Day 5 Lunch
  » Wild Rice Power Bowl—Day 5 Dinner

- If you have a busy schedule, you could prepare a larger batch of each soup at the start of the week and freeze or refrigerate portions.

- Orange and Spice Overnight Oats and Tropical Chia Pudding should be prepped the night before.

- You'll be storing multiple soups and dishes at once, so plan your fridge/freezer space.

Phase 2 Daily Checklist

MORNING

- ○ 2 glasses water
- ○ Morning supplements at <u>scheduled</u> time
  - ◉ Low FODMAP prebiotic supplement (start low, go slow) (see cheat sheet, page 173)
  - ◉ Vitamin D (see cheat sheet, page 179)
  - ◉ Omega-3 (see cheat sheet, page 181)
  - ◉ Turmeric supplement (see cheat sheet, page 189)
- ○ 30 minutes sunlight
- ○ 30 minutes of light exercise, preferably outdoors *NEW*
- ○ 3–5 minutes breathwork training

EVENING

- ○ No caffeine or carbonated drinks
- ○ No solid food after 8:00 p.m.
- ○ Minimize light exposure: dim lighting, blue light filters, digital detox
- ○ Evening supplements at <u>scheduled</u> time
  - ◉ Melatonin supplement (see cheat sheet, page 182)
  - ◉ Zinc supplement (see cheat sheet, page 185)
  - ◉ Magnesium supplement (see cheat sheet, page 184)
- ○ 3–5 minutes breathwork
- ○ Consistent bedtime
- ○ 7–8 hours in bed

LIFESTYLE

- ○ Start a 14-hour time-restricted eating pattern (14 hours fasting, 10 hours feeding). *NEW*
- ○ Resistance training exercise at least 3X this week *NEW*
- ○ No alcohol, tobacco, or marijuana

○ Turn off phone at mealtimes.
○ Limit time spent on social media and devices, aiming for meaningful in-person interactions instead. *NEW*
○ Use mealtimes to connect with others. *NEW*

PHASE 2 HOMEWORK (DO ONCE THIS PHASE)

○ Practice forgiveness and let go of resentment to reduce emotional and physiological stress. This might include a strained relationship with a close family member or friend. *NEW*
○ Embrace a growth mindset. Begin to reappraise difficult life events as opportunities for growth rather than setbacks. *NEW*
○ If there is trauma or something more serious impacting your emotional health, schedule an appointment with a health professional. *NEW*
○ Take a step toward spiritual health. This can be as big or as small as you feel comfortable with. Examples include spending time in prayer or quiet reflection, reading from religious scripture, or attending a service. *NEW*
○ Take a weekly 15-minute "awe walk" to appreciate nature and spark a sense of wonder.

EXTRA CREDIT

○ Visit your local farmers' market. *NEW*
○ Try sprouting at home. *NEW*
○ Consider adding a targeted probiotic supplement if needed. *NEW*
○ Explore acts of service or volunteer opportunities to enhance spiritual purpose. *NEW*

PHASE 3: MASTERY

Goals: Gut-immune optimization,
empowered gut health, building resilience

Phase 3: Mastery is where all the effort and dedication from the earlier phases culminates in thriving health and resilience. This is the phase of optimization—fine-tuning your habits, exploring advanced strategies, and achieving a deeper connection to your gut-immune health. In this phase, you'll focus on maintaining and expanding what you've built, integrating even more diversity into your diet and enhancing your life-style practices for sustained vitality. It's about creating a life where you feel empowered, energetic, and resilient, fully equipped to navigate challenges while continuing to grow. **Mastery** is not about perfection but about living in alignment with your health goals and thriving every step of the way.

The recipes for **Phase 3** include five breakfasts, ten entrées, two soups, three beverages, and three snacks or desserts. This is a build on the recipes from **Growth**, so you have the freedom to piece together what works for you. Once again, on a daily basis you will build out your meal plan to include one breakfast followed by the entrées or soup for lunch and dinner. The beverages, snacks, and desserts are added as desired. Continue your daily smoothie habit.

Phase 3 Nutrition Guidelines

Prioritize	30+ different plants per week *UPDATED*
	90+ percent whole foods (10 percent or less ultra-processed foods) *UPDATED*
	Fermented foods twice daily *UPDATED*
	Start to introduce high FODMAP plant-based foods and raw vegetables *NEW*
	Make sure to get varied colors among your plant foods, for more polyphenol variety
Allowed	Low FODMAP protein powder (plain brown rice protein or a certified low FODMAP protein) in smoothies if skipping breakfast
	Extra-virgin olive oil
	If consuming animal products, prioritize fish and shellfish, fermented dairy, and eggs.
	Sourdough bread (if tolerating gluten)
Off-Limits	Added sugar or artificial sweeteners except fermented drinks (stevia and monk fruit are okay)
	Gluten and flour except sourdough
	Salty snacks
	Fried foods
	Sugary desserts or candy
	Processed meats
	Fast food

Phase 3 Weekly Meal Plan

DAY 1		
BREAKFAST	**LUNCH**	**DINNER**
Avocado Toast with a Dukkah Twist	15-Minute Tortilla Soup	Crunchy Tempeh Tacos

DAY 2		
BREAKFAST	**LUNCH**	**DINNER**
Peanut Pumpkin Power Bowl	Crunchy Tempeh Tacos (leftovers from Day 1)	Southwest Quinoa Salad with Cumin Lime Dressing

DAY 3

BREAKFAST	LUNCH	DINNER
Avocado Toast with a Dukkah Twist	Eat the Rainbow Salad	Mulligatawny Soup

DAY 4

BREAKFAST	LUNCH	DINNER
Morning Sundae Surprise	Mulligatawny Soup (leftovers from Day 3)	Citrus Kale Pasta Salad

DAY 5

BREAKFAST	LUNCH	DINNER
Speedy Chickpea Shakshuka	Double Strawberry Spring Salad	Spiced Chickpea and Beet Yogurt Bowl

DAY 6

BREAKFAST	LUNCH	DINNER
Cherry Pie Chia Pudding	Hummus Kimchi Wraps	Forbidden Rice Salad

DAY 7

BREAKFAST	LUNCH	DINNER
Speedy Chickpea Shakshuka (leftovers from Day 5)	Springtime Panzanella Salad	Pre and Pro Miso Bowl

Phase 3 Optional Recipes

SMOOTHIES	SNACKS AND SWEETS	BEVERAGES	PROTEIN ADD-ONS
Start your morning with a smoothie.	Listen to your hunger cues between lunch and dinner.	Add polyphenol-rich beverages throughout the day.	Flexible proteins to add as desired to your meals.
Top Secret Mango Lassi (page 325) *NEW* Spiced Pomegranate Lassi (page 326) *NEW*	Smoked Chili Lime Popcorn (page 361) *NEW* Cashew Citrus Energy Bites (page 357) *NEW*	Summer Garden Blended Juice (page 324) *NEW* Ginger Green Refresher (page 278)	Crispy Baked Tofu (page 362) The *Best* Tempeh (page 363)

Golden Green Kickstart Smoothie (page 281)	Chocolate-Drizzled Berry Bites (page 359)	Citrus-Spiced Golden Milk (page 279)	Soft/Medium/ Hard-Boiled Eggs
Citrus Berry Belly Bliss Smoothie (page 282)	*NEW*	The Blue Zen Elixir (page 280)	(page 365)
	Fruits		Easy Pan-Seared Salmon (page 366)
	Nuts	Tropic Mint Kiwi Cooler (page 283)	Stovetop Shrimp
	Smoothie		(page 367)
	Berries	Green and black tea	
	Dark Chocolate	Herbal tea	
		Coffee	
		Kombucha	

WEEK 3 PLANT TOTAL: 60 UNIQUE PLANTS

NOTES ON PHASE 3 MEAL PLAN:

- If you'd like a shopping list for Phase 3, head to my website—www .theguthealthmd.com/plantpoweredplus.

- To make 1 batch of 15-Minute Tortilla Soup (4 cups), Mulligatawny Soup (4 cups), and the Pre and Pro Miso Bowl (4 cups), you'll need 12 cups of P3 Biome Broth. Or you can make 10 cups of P3 Biome Broth and stretch it with water.

- If you have a busy schedule, you could prepare a larger batch of each soup at the start of the week and freeze or refrigerate portions. Also feel free to pair the leftover soup with a salad or the kimchi wraps.

- You'll be storing multiple leftovers and possibly big batches of broth. Label containers with dates so you don't mix them up.

- The Cherry Pie Chia Pudding benefits from chilling. Consider prepping it the night before.

Phase 3 Daily Checklist

MORNING

- ○ 2 glasses water
- ○ Morning supplements at <u>scheduled</u> time
  - ○ Low FODMAP prebiotic supplement (start low, go slow) (see cheat sheet, page 173)
  - ○ Vitamin D (increase if appropriate) (see cheat sheet, page 179)
  - ○ Omega-3 (increase if appropriate) (see cheat sheet, page 181)
  - ○ Turmeric supplement (increase if appropriate) (see cheat sheet, page 189)
- ○ 30 minutes of sunlight
- ○ 30 minutes of light exercise, preferably outdoors
- ○ 3–5 minutes breathwork training

EVENING

- ○ No caffeine or carbonated drinks
- ○ No solid food after 8:00 p.m.
- ○ Minimize light exposure: dim lighting, blue light filters, digital detox
- ○ Evening supplements at <u>scheduled</u> time
  - ○ Melatonin supplement (see cheat sheet, page 182)
  - ○ Zinc supplement (see cheat sheet, page 185)
  - ○ Magnesium supplement (see cheat sheet, page 184)
- ○ 3–5 minutes breathwork
- ○ Add a calming activity like meditation, aromatherapy, gentle stretching, or prayer to prepare for restful sleep. *NEW*
- ○ Consistent bedtime
- ○ 7–8 hours in bed

LIFESTYLE

○ Increase to 16-hour time-restricted eating pattern (16 hours fasting, 8 hours feeding). *UPDATED*

⬤ Maintain regular mealtimes. *NEW*

○ Resistance training exercise at least 4X this week *UPDATED*

⬤ Experiment with exercise timing to find the best time for you. *NEW*

○ No alcohol, tobacco, or marijuana

○ Develop a consistent spiritual practice, including daily prayer, meditation, and reading from scripture. *NEW*

○ Turn off phone at mealtimes.

○ Limit time spent on social media and devices, aiming for meaningful in-person interactions instead.

○ Use mealtimes to connect with others.

PHASE 3 HOMEWORK (DO ONCE THIS PHASE)

○ Strengthen your closest connection. Dedicate intentional time to your partner or a trusted friend, connecting on something important and deeply personal to you. *NEW*

○ If you have a strained relationship with a close family member or friend, reach out and reconnect with that person. *NEW*

○ Cultivate a purpose-driven life. Reflect deeply on personal values and pursue activities aligned with a greater purpose. *NEW*

○ Plan a trip to an awe-inspiring location and take a 15-minute "awe walk" to appreciate nature and spark a sense of wonder. Tag me @theguthealthmd when you do. *UPDATED*

EXTRA CREDIT

○ Create a sourdough starter. *NEW*

○ Make your own sauerkraut, kimchi, pickles, or dilly beans. *NEW*

○ Start an herb garden at home. *NEW*

○ Work with a professional to address unresolved trauma through methods like EMDR or trauma-focused therapy. *NEW*

○ Use advanced tracking to fine-tune sleep habits. Monitor heart rate variability (HRV) or sleep quality. *NEW*

○ Repeat blood work and refine supplement levels. *NEW*

○ Expand social bonds. Mentor or support others on their journey. Foster intergenerational connections through family or community involvement. *NEW*

What to Do When You Finish Phase 3?

As a part of my books, I appreciate the opportunity to share some parting thoughts and encouragement. Head over to page 369 in the Epilogue for closing reflections and next steps on your journey.

Ginger Green Refresher

4 PLANT POINTS

Greens are the most nutrient-dense foods that exist, and we want to make the most of that with this green juice recipe that incorporates gut-nurturing ginger and citrus for the vitamin C. Green juices are fantastic for healing; I just hate when we separate out the fiber and discard it. So we won't do that. Instead, we'll blend our juice and get the best of both worlds.

SERVES 1
TOTAL TIME: 5 MINUTES

---

1 cup lightly packed baby arugula

6 green grapes

1 inch peeled and chopped fresh ginger

2 tablespoons lemon juice (about 1½ small lemons)

1. Combine the arugula, grapes, ginger, lemon juice, and 2 cups water in a blender and blend until smooth.

2. Pour over ice to serve.

Pro Tip
To make ahead, triple the recipe and store it in a sealed mason jar or other container for up to 4 days.

Citrus-Spiced Golden Milk

5 PLANT POINTS

Warm up your gut with this soothing, citrus-infused golden milk. Fresh orange juice, ginger, and turmeric bring bright, spicy notes and an anti-inflammatory boost to every sip. Perfect for a cozy morning treat or an evening wind-down, this golden milk is just what your doctor and dietitian ordered!

SERVES 1
TOTAL TIME: 5 MINUTES

1½ cups almond milk (or other low FODMAP plant-based milk)

1 medium orange, zested and juiced (about 3 tablespoons juice)

1 teaspoon 100% maple syrup or to taste

¾ teaspoon ground turmeric

½ teaspoon ground ginger

Freshly ground black pepper to taste (optional)

1. Heat the almond milk in a microwave-safe cup for approximately 2 minutes. Or bring it to a boil on the stovetop in a small saucepan over high heat.

2. Carefully pour the hot liquid into a blender. Add the orange juice, maple syrup, turmeric, and ginger. Cover and blend until frothy.

3. Pour into a mug, top with orange zest and pepper, and enjoy.

The Blue Zen Elixir

3 PLANT POINTS

Indulge in a gentle blend of fragrant lavender, zesty lemon, and sweet blueberries in this soothing elixir. Whether you savor it chilled for an afternoon refreshment or warmed for a calming bedtime bevvy, this aromatic drink is ready to nourish and hydrate any time of day.

SERVES 4
TOTAL TIME: 35 MINUTES

1 cup frozen blueberries (ideally organic and wild)

1 tablespoon culinary-grade lavender

1 lemon, zested and juiced

4 cups boiling water

1. Place the blueberries, lavender, and lemon zest in a medium to large heatproof pitcher. Carefully pour the hot water into the pitcher and steep for 30 minutes. Add the lemon juice to the mixture.

2. Strain into a mug to enjoy hot. Or place the pitcher in the refrigerator to serve cold.

Pro Tip
Combine with sparkling water for a delicious low-sugar mocktail. To make ahead, double or triple the batch and store in the refrigerator for up to 1 week.

Golden Green Kickstart Smoothie

5 PLANT POINTS

If you're looking for a belly-friendly anti-inflammatory smoothie, you'll love this refreshing Golden Green Kickstart Smoothie. The pineapple's sweet and tangy flavor pairs perfectly with ginger's spicy kick, while the arugula adds a nutrient super boost. Add your favorite protein powder, if desired, for a complete meal.

SERVES 1
TOTAL TIME: 5 MINUTES

1 cup almond milk or other low FODMAP plant-based milk

½ medium orange, peeled, seeds removed, and cut into quarters

¾ cup frozen pineapple

1 cup arugula or other low FODMAP leafy greens

½ teaspoon ground ginger

Optional: Add 1 teaspoon 100% maple syrup or to taste, a pinch of salt, and/or low FODMAP protein powder.

1. Place the almond milk, orange pieces, pineapple, arugula, and ginger in a blender. Add the maple syrup, a pinch of salt, and/or protein powder if desired. Blend on high speed until smooth.

2. Pour into a glass and enjoy.

Pro Tip
Low FODMAP protein powder options: Choose plain brown rice protein or a certified low FODMAP protein powder.

Citrus Berry Belly Bliss Smoothie

5 PLANT POINTS

This Citrus Berry Belly Bliss Smoothie (say that five times fast) is powered by all four workhorses, including yogurt, ginger, and flaxseeds. You'll check all four boxes in one delicious drink. Strawberries and oranges offer natural sweetness with no sugar added. This is what winning looks like!

SERVES 1
TOTAL TIME: 5 MINUTES

---

1 cup almond milk or other low FODMAP plant-based milk

½ cup plain unsweetened almond milk yogurt

1 whole orange, zested, peeled, and cut into quarters

5 frozen or fresh (hulled) strawberries

1 tablespoon ground flaxseed

½ teaspoon ground ginger

Optional: Add 1 teaspoon 100% maple syrup, a pinch of salt, and low FODMAP protein powder (see Pro Tip on page 281 for options).

1. Place the almond milk, yogurt, orange pieces, strawberries, flaxseed, and ginger in a blender. Add the maple syrup, a pinch of salt, and/or protein powder if desired. Blend on high speed until smooth.

2. Pour into a glass, top with orange zest, and enjoy.

Pro Tip
Swap the strawberries with frozen or fresh polyphenol-rich cranberries when they are readily available in the fall and winter.

Tropic Mint Kiwi Cooler

5 PLANT POINTS

A burst of sweet-tart flavor from the kiwi (you know I love kiwis bursting, as seen on the covers of my previous two books!) pairs perfectly with fresh mint and creamy almond milk, while a sprinkle of shredded coconut adds a hint of tropical flair. Enjoy this hydrating drink anytime you crave a cool, revitalizing treat.

SERVES 1
TOTAL TIME: 5 MINUTES

½ cup almond milk

⅓ cup coconut water

2 kiwifruit, peeled

¼ to ½ cup lightly packed fresh mint leaves

1 lime, zested and juiced

1 teaspoon shredded unsweetened coconut

1. Place the almond milk, coconut water, kiwifruit, mint leaves, and lime juice in a blender. Blend on high speed until smooth.

2. Pour into a glass over ice, top with shredded coconut and lime zest, and enjoy.

Oatmeal Cookie Dough Smoothie

6 PLANT POINTS

When the craving for oatmeal cookies hits, reach for this dreamy, naturally sweetened Oatmeal Cookie Dough Smoothie. Raw oats provide gut microbiome–friendly resistant starch, while walnuts add creaminess and omega-3s.

SERVES 1
TOTAL TIME: 5 MINUTES

¾ cup almond milk

½ cup gluten-free oats (organic)

¼ cup raw walnuts

1 small pitted Medjool date

½ teaspoon ground cinnamon, plus more for topping

2 or 3 ice cubes

1 teaspoon raisins

Optional: Add a pinch of salt and low FODMAP protein powder (see Pro Tip on page 281 for options).

1. Place the almond milk, oats, walnuts, date, cinnamon, and ice in a blender. Add the salt and/or protein powder if desired. Blend on high speed until smooth.

2. Pour into a glass over ice, top with raisins and cinnamon, and enjoy.

P3 Biome Broth

9 PLANT POINTS

Many people with gut or autoimmune issues turn to soothing bone broth, but bones transfer toxic heavy metals when heated. EEEK! Instead, let's center our broth around anti-inflammatory plants. Store-bought broths often rely on onions and garlic—problematic for those on a low FODMAP diet—while this homemade version swaps in aromatic herbs, savory mushrooms, and colorful vegetables to create a rich, comforting base without high FODMAP ingredients. Enjoy it as a cozy sipper, or use it to add depth and nutrition to soups, sauces, and beyond for fuss-free, flavorful cooking.

SERVES 10
TOTAL TIME: 1 HOUR 10 MINUTES (10 MINUTES ACTIVE TIME)

---

2 cups roughly chopped carrots

2 cored tomatoes, quartered

1 cup roughly chopped parsnips

1 cup sliced leeks, green part only

1 cup sliced green onion tops

1 stalk celery, roughly chopped

1 cup oyster mushrooms

5 sprigs fresh thyme

1 teaspoon black peppercorns

1. Add the carrots, tomatoes, parsnips, leek greens, green onions, celery, mushrooms, thyme, and peppercorns to a large stockpot. Cover with 10 cups water.

2. Cover the pot and bring to a boil over high heat, then reduce the heat to low and simmer for 1 hour. Remove from the heat and let cool.

recipe continues

3. After the stock has cooled, strain the broth through a fine-mesh strainer and transfer it to refrigerator- or freezer-safe glass jars or containers.

4. Seal the containers well and store them in the refrigerator for up to 4 days or in the freezer (allow extra room for expansion) for up to 6 months.

Sun-Kissed Curry Carrot Soup

10 PLANT POINTS

Brightly spiced with curry and ginger, this creamy carrot soup harnesses the power of cooked-and-cooled potatoes for added resistant starch. Infused with citrusy orange and finished with a dollop of yogurt and cilantro, each spoonful bursts with flavor and gut-friendly benefits.

SERVES 5

TOTAL TIME: 40 MINUTES (15 MINUTES ACTIVE TIME)

1½ cups diced white or yellow (e.g., Yukon Gold) potatoes

1 tablespoon extra-virgin olive oil

1 teaspoon garlic-infused oil

3 cups finely chopped carrots

2 teaspoons curry powder

1 teaspoon peeled and minced fresh ginger

½ teaspoon salt or to taste

Freshly ground black pepper to taste

4 cups P3 Biome Broth (page 285) or water

1 orange, zested and juiced

5 tablespoons almond milk yogurt or other low FODMAP yogurt

5 tablespoons chopped cilantro

Optional: Add a sprinkle of hempseeds, chia seeds, and/or pumpkin seeds for extra protein, fiber, and healthy fats!

1. Add the potatoes to a medium saucepan and add along with enough water to cover. Bring to a boil over high heat, then reduce the heat to low and cook the potatoes for 10 minutes, or until tender. Drain and place the potatoes in a freezer-safe container in the freezer to quickly cool.

recipe continues

2. Heat the olive oil and garlic oil in a medium to large pot over medium heat. Add the carrots and sauté for 2 minutes. Stir in the curry powder, ginger, salt, and pepper and sauté for 2 minutes.

3. Add the broth to the pot along with the orange juice and zest and cooled potatoes. Bring to a boil, reduce the heat to low, and simmer for 5 minutes.

4. Carefully pour the soup into a blender and blend it on high speed until it is smooth. Taste and add additional salt and/or pepper if desired.

5. Divide into 5 bowls to serve and top each bowl with yogurt and cilantro.

6. Store the soup in an airtight container in the refrigerator for up to 4 days or in the freezer (allow room in the container for expansion) for up to 4 months.

Creamy Cannellini and Parsnip Soup

6 PLANT POINTS

Fresh rosemary and tender leek greens infuse each spoonful with bright herbal notes, while a quick whirl in the blender brings the parsnips and cannellini beans together into a velvety bowl of goodness.

SERVES 6

TOTAL TIME: 45 MINUTES (15 MINUTES ACTIVE TIME)

1 tablespoon extra-virgin olive oil

1 teaspoon garlic-infused oil

1½ cups sliced leeks, green part only

1 pound parsnips, peeled and diced

2 teaspoons finely chopped fresh rosemary

¾ teaspoon salt or to taste

Freshly ground black pepper to taste

6 cups P3 Biome Broth (page 285) or water

One 15-ounce can cannellini beans, rinsed and drained

1. Heat the olive oil and garlic oil in a large stockpot over medium heat. Add the leeks and sauté for 5 minutes to soften.

2. Add the parsnips, rosemary, salt, and pepper to the pot and stir well to combine.

3. Add the broth to the pot. Bring to a boil over high heat, then reduce the heat to low and simmer for 15 minutes. Add the beans, raise the heat to medium, and cook for 5 more minutes.

recipe continues

4. Carefully pour the soup into a blender and blend it on high speed until it is smooth. Taste and add additional salt and/or pepper if desired before serving.

5. Store the soup in an airtight container in the refrigerator for up to 4 days or in the freezer (allow room in the container for expansion) for up to 6 months.

Citrus-Kissed Cannellini Stew

10 PLANT POINTS

Savor the bright tang of fresh lemon in this nourishing soup featuring hearty buckwheat groats and creamy cannellini beans—perfect for a light lunch or a comforting dinner.

SERVES 6

TOTAL TIME: 45 MINUTES (25 MINUTES ACTIVE TIME)

1 tablespoon extra-virgin olive oil

1 teaspoon garlic-infused oil

1½ cups sliced leeks, green part only

2 cups finely chopped carrots

1 cup diced zucchini

1 teaspoon smoked paprika

1 tablespoon chopped fresh oregano, or 1 teaspoon dried, plus more for garnish

1½ teaspoons salt or to taste

Freshly ground black pepper to taste

6 cups P3 Biome Broth (page 285) or water

1 cup buckwheat groats

One 15-ounce can cannellini beans, rinsed and drained

2 lemons, cut into quarters

1. Heat a large stockpot over medium heat. Add the olive oil, garlic oil, and leeks to the pot. Sauté for 2 minutes.

2. Add the carrots and zucchini and sauté for 2 minutes.

3. Stir in the paprika, oregano, salt, and pepper.

4. Pour the broth over the vegetables. Cover and bring to a boil over high heat, then add the buckwheat. Reduce the heat to low and cook for 10 minutes.

recipe continues

5. Add the beans and cook for 3 more minutes.

6. To serve: Divide the soup into 6 bowls. Serve with lemon wedges and garnish with additional fresh oregano if desired.

7. Store the soup in an airtight container in the refrigerator for up to 4 days or in the freezer (allow room in the container for expansion) for up to 6 months.

Pro Tip
Swap fresh or dried thyme in place of oregano or use quinoa instead of buckwheat.

Rosemary Minestrone Soup

12 PLANT POINTS

I'm a lifelong fan of minestrone soup. Plain and simple, start with a tasty, herbal base and then just start throwing plants in. The more the merrier. The flavors meld, and next thing you know both you and your microbes are feasting joyfully. Add a sprinkle of crushed red pepper flakes to kick it up a notch.

SERVES 4

TOTAL TIME: 45 MINUTES (30 MINUTES ACTIVE TIME)

1½ cups dried chickpea pasta (e.g., elbows or shells)

1 tablespoon extra-virgin olive oil

1 teaspoon garlic-infused oil

1½ cups sliced leeks, green part only

1½ cups diced carrots

1 stalk celery, thinly sliced

1 tablespoon fresh rosemary, or 1 teaspoon dried

1½ teaspoons dried oregano

1½ teaspoons dried thyme

1¼ teaspoons salt or to taste

Freshly ground black pepper to taste

2 cups canned diced tomatoes with juice

3 cups P3 Biome Broth (page 285) or water

1⅓ cups canned cannellini beans, rinsed and drained

One 10-ounce bag frozen cut green beans

Crushed red pepper flakes to taste (optional)

1. Cook the pasta according to package directions.

2. Heat the olive oil and garlic oil in a large pot over medium-high heat. Add the leeks and sauté for 3 minutes. Add the carrots and celery and sauté for 2 or 3 more minutes.

recipe continues

3. Season the vegetables with the rosemary, oregano, thyme, salt, and pepper.

4. Add the tomatoes, broth, cannellini beans, and green beans to the pot and stir until combined. Bring the soup to a boil, reduce the heat to low, and simmer for 10 minutes.

5. Drain the cooked pasta, then add 3 cups to the soup. Season with additional salt and pepper if desired.

6. Divide the soup among 4 bowls and serve with red pepper flakes, if using.

7. Store the soup in an airtight container in the refrigerator for up to 4 days or in the freezer (allow room in the container for expansion) for up to 6 months.

Orange and Spice Overnight Oats

8 PLANT POINTS

If you haven't paired orange and cardamom before, you're in for a delicious treat! This recipe is easy to prep the night before—set it and forget it—then enjoy it in the morning.

SERVES 2

TOTAL TIME: 40 MINUTES (10 MINUTES ACTIVE TIME)

⅔ cup gluten-free oats (organic)

2 tablespoons ground flaxseed

½ teaspoon ground ginger

¼ teaspoon ground cardamom

⅛ teaspoon salt (optional)

1 cup unsweetened almond milk

1 teaspoon vanilla extract

2 teaspoons 100% maple syrup or to taste

2 small to medium oranges, peeled and cut into ½-inch pieces

½ cup sliced raw almonds

Optional: Top with lactose-free plain unsweetened kefir for a low FODMAP vegetarian version.

1. Combine the oats, flaxseed, ginger, cardamom, and salt, if using, in a bowl. Stir well to combine.

2. Add the almond milk, vanilla, and maple syrup to the mixture and stir to combine.

3. Divide the mixture into 2 serving bowls or small mason jars. Refrigerate for at least 30 minutes or overnight.

4. To serve: Top each serving with orange pieces and sliced almonds.

5. Store in the refrigerator for up to 4 days.

Wild Blueberry Chia Crisp with Yogurt

8 PLANT POINTS

This Wild Blueberry Chia Crisp is healthy for breakfast and delicious enough to enjoy for dessert! You'll love this easy recipe featuring whole-grain gluten-free oats, omega-3-rich chia seeds, polyphenol-rich wild blueberries, and anti-inflammatory-rich ginger. Add a scoop of yogurt and you'll have all four workhorses on board!

SERVES 4
TOTAL TIME: 35 MINUTES (10 MINUTES ACTIVE TIME)

3 cups frozen wild blueberries (preferably organic, no need to thaw)

¼ cup chia seeds

3 tablespoons 100% maple syrup

2 tablespoons tapioca flour

½ teaspoon ground ginger

⅛ teaspoon salt (optional)

3 tablespoons avocado oil

¾ cup gluten-free oats (organic)

¼ cup sorghum flour

1 cup almond yogurt (or lactose-free plain yogurt)

Optional: Top with slivered almonds or chopped walnuts for extra crunch!

1. Preheat the oven to 350°F.

2. Combine the blueberries, chia seeds, 1 tablespoon of the maple syrup, the tapioca flour, ginger, and salt, if using, in a medium bowl. Stir well to combine, ensuring that all of the blueberries are coated with chia seeds and flour.

3. Divide the blueberries into 4 custard cups or oven-safe ramekins and place them on a baking sheet.

4. Add the avocado oil, remaining 2 tablespoons of maple syrup, oats, and flour to the bowl and stir well to combine.

5. Divide the topping evenly over the blueberry mixture and bake for 20 to 25 minutes, until lightly browned.

6. Remove from the oven, cool, and top each serving with ¼ cup yogurt.

Pro Tip

All blueberries are rich in polyphenols; however, wild blueberries have the highest amount. If you can't find wild blueberries in your grocery store, swap them with regular frozen blueberries. Brown rice flour can be used in place of the sorghum flour.

Tropical Chia Pudding

8 PLANT POINTS

Take your taste buds on vacation to the tropics with this creamy Tropical Chia Pudding. The great thing is that your gut may be on vacation, but you won't have vacation gut. Chia seeds and kiwifruit help with regularity while being gentle on your digestive tract.

SERVES 4
TOTAL TIME: 30 MINUTES (15 MINUTES ACTIVE TIME)

2 cups frozen pineapple chunks

½ cup chia seeds

½ cup light coconut milk

½ cup almond milk

2 tablespoons 100% maple syrup

1 teaspoon vanilla extract

⅛ teaspoon salt

½ cup slivered raw almonds

4 kiwifruit, peeled and diced

½ cup fresh mint, for garnish

1. Thaw the pineapple in the refrigerator, or heat it for 1 to 2 minutes in the microwave.

2. Combine the chia seeds, coconut milk, almond milk, maple syrup, vanilla, and salt in a medium bowl. Stir well to combine the ingredients. Stir every 5 minutes for the first 10 minutes to keep the mixture from clumping, then place in the refrigerator for 20 minutes, or until the pudding has thickened.

3. To serve: Spread a layer of chia pudding in 4 serving dishes. Top with pineapple and 1 tablespoon of almonds on each serving. Add another layer of chia pudding, then top with

the kiwifruit and the remaining almonds. Garnish with
fresh mint.

4. Store in the refrigerator for up to 4 days.

Pro Tip
Try macadamia nuts in place of the almonds for a super-tropical kick!

Kimchi Tofu Scramble Breakfast Tacos

9 PLANT POINTS

Scrambled tofu is a tasty plant-based protein swap for eggs in these flavorful breakfast tacos, which feature probiotic-rich kimchi, creamy avocado, and your daily dose of leafy greens. They deliver big flavor in minimal time—perfect for busy mornings.

SERVES 2
TOTAL TIME: 10 MINUTES

1 tablespoon extra-virgin olive oil

8 ounces firm tofu (organic), crumbled

2 cups lightly packed baby spinach, roughly chopped

¼ cup kimchi

1 teaspoon gluten-free tamari

1 teaspoon toasted sesame oil

4 corn tortillas

6 tablespoons mashed avocado

½ cup sliced green onion tops

½ cup lightly packed fresh cilantro, roughly chopped

Optional: You can use regular scrambled eggs if you prefer.

1. Heat the olive oil in a medium to large skillet over medium-high heat. Add the tofu to the pan and sauté for 2 minutes. Add the spinach and sauté for 1 minute.

2. Stir in the kimchi, tamari, and sesame oil, then transfer the tofu mixture to a medium bowl.

3. Wipe the skillet, then heat the tortillas, 2 at a time, over medium-high heat until soft and warm.

4. To serve: Spread 1½ tablespoons of avocado on each tortilla, then divide the tofu mixture among the 4 tortillas. Top each taco with green onions and cilantro.

Pro Tip

Cook a big batch of scrambled tofu ahead of time and store it in the refrigerator in a well-sealed container for up to 4 days.

Cinnamon Crunch Buckwheat Granola

8 PLANT POINTS

Crunchy oats and nutty buckwheat groats come together in this lightly sweet, cinnamon-spiced granola. As an added bonus, oats and buckwheat are both sources of gut-friendly resistant starch. We love that. Prep time is only 10 minutes. Eat it as is, or serve over your favorite yogurt or smoothie bowl with some berries.

SERVES 9
TOTAL TIME: 35 MINUTES (10 MINUTES ACTIVE TIME)

2 cups gluten-free oats (organic)

1 cup buckwheat groats

½ cup raw pecans, chopped

½ cup raw walnuts, chopped

½ cup sunflower seeds

2½ teaspoons ground cinnamon

¼ to ½ teaspoon salt or to taste

½ cup avocado oil

½ cup plus 2 tablespoons 100% maple syrup

Optional: Serve with almond milk or lactose-free plain unsweetened kefir.

1. Preheat the oven to 325°F. Line a large baking sheet with parchment paper.

2. Combine the oats, buckwheat, pecans, walnuts, sunflower seeds, cinnamon, and salt in a large bowl. Stir well to mix the ingredients together.

3. Add the avocado oil and maple syrup to the oat mixture, stirring to coat all the oats.

4. Spread the granola evenly on the parchment-lined baking sheet and bake for 10 minutes. Stir the granola, then spread it on the sheet again, pressing down on the mixture.

5. Bake for 10 more minutes, then remove the granola from the oven and allow it to cool completely. For clumpier granola, press down on the mixture after removing it from the oven and before thoroughly cooling it.

6. Break the granola into pieces and store it in a well-sealed container at room temperature for up to 1 week or in the freezer for up to 4 months.

Wild Blueberry Smoothie Bowl

7 PLANT POINTS

This big beautiful blueberry smoothie bowl is packed with so much goodness! Ready in minutes, it's the perfect anytime refresh.

SERVES 1
TOTAL TIME: 10 MINUTES

½ cup almond milk

1 cup frozen wild blueberries (preferably organic)

1 tablespoon ground flaxseed

¼ teaspoon ground ginger

Pinch of salt (optional)

⅓ cup Cinnamon Crunch Buckwheat Granola (page 302)

1 kiwifruit, peeled and sliced

1 tablespoon hempseeds

Optional: Use low FODMAP protein powder and edible flowers to garnish. The almond milk can be replaced with lactose-free plain unsweetened kefir for extra protein and probiotics.

1. Add the almond milk, blueberries, flaxseed, ginger, and salt, if using, to a blender. Blend on high speed to combine the ingredients. Add optional protein powder if desired. You may also add additional almond milk if needed for a thinner consistency.

2. Pour the smoothie into a serving bowl. Top with granola, kiwi slices, hempseeds, and optional edible flowers.

Easy Stir-Fried Veggie and Edamame Rice

9 PLANT POINTS

Put your freezer to work by making this delicious stir-fried rice with frozen brown rice, corn, and edamame. Broccoli, carrots, garlic oil, sesame oil, soy sauce, and green onions round out the flavors in this healthy comfort-food dish!

SERVES 4
TOTAL TIME: 20 MINUTES

2 tablespoons avocado oil

3 to 4 roughly chopped carrots (about 1 cup)

1 cup roughly chopped broccoli crown

Salt and freshly ground black pepper to taste

4 cups frozen precooked brown rice

2 cups frozen edamame

1 cup frozen corn

1 tablespoon low-sodium gluten-free tamari or to taste

1 teaspoon garlic-infused oil

1 teaspoon toasted sesame oil

1 cup sliced green onion tops

Optional: In addition to the green onions, other delicious toppings include sesame seeds, pine nuts, and fresh cilantro. Top with approximately 3 ounces per each serving Stovetop Shrimp (page 367) for a pescatarian version.

1. Heat the avocado oil in a wok or large frying pan over medium-high heat. Add the carrots and broccoli and sauté them for 3 minutes, or until lightly softened. Season with salt and pepper.

recipe continues

2. Stir in the frozen rice, edamame, and corn. Stir for about 5 minutes, or until the rice and vegetables are cooked.

3. Remove from the heat and stir in the tamari, garlic oil, and sesame oil.

4. Divide into 4 servings and top each serving with ¼ cup green onions.

Pro Tip

This recipe tastes even better the next day, so double it if needed to enjoy for leftovers. Store the fried rice in an airtight container in the refrigerator for up to 4 days.

Miso-Licious Vegetable Pasta

7 PLANT POINTS

Give your pasta night a savory twist with miso-roasted broccoli, carrots, and bell peppers. A quick whisk of miso and olive oil turns ordinary veggies into an umami-rich centerpiece, while chickpea pasta and pine nuts bring satisfying protein and crunch.

SERVES 4

TOTAL TIME: 45 MINUTES (15 MINUTES ACTIVE TIME)

2 tablespoons miso

6 tablespoons extra-virgin olive oil

3 cups bite-sized broccoli crown florets

2 cups sliced carrots (about 4 medium carrots)

1 cup diced red bell pepper (about ½ large pepper)

One 8-ounce package of chickpea rotini pasta

¼ cup raw pine nuts

Salt and freshly ground black pepper to taste

Crushed red pepper flakes to taste (optional)

1 cup chopped fresh flat-leaf parsley, for garnish (optional)

Optional: If desired, add a piece of Easy Pan-Seared Salmon (page 366) over the top or Stovetop Shrimp (page 367) on top.

1. Preheat the oven to 425°F. Line a baking sheet with parchment paper or aluminum foil.

2. Add the miso to a medium or large bowl with 1 tablespoon water and whisk to soften the miso. Stir in 2 tablespoons of the olive oil, then add the broccoli, carrots, and bell pepper. Stir the vegetables to coat them with the miso–olive oil mixture, then spread them out on the parchment-lined baking sheet and bake for 20 minutes.

recipe continues

3. Cook the pasta according to the package directions while the vegetables are roasting. Drain the cooked pasta and place it in a serving bowl.

4. Add the roasted vegetables and pine nuts to the pasta. Top with the remaining 4 tablespoons of olive oil and season with salt and pepper. Stir well to combine the ingredients.

5. Divide the pasta among 4 serving dishes and garnish with red pepper flakes and parsley, if using.

Herby Chickpea Quinoa Salad

11 PLANT POINTS

This Mediterranean-inspired chickpea quinoa salad is a crowd favorite! Make a big batch ahead of time for a quick and easy light lunch or dinner. Feel free to use your favorite combination of fresh and dried herbs.

SERVES 4

TOTAL TIME: 25 MINUTES (10 MINUTES ACTIVE TIME)

1 cup quinoa, rinsed

1 large cucumber, peeled and diced

2 medium tomatoes, diced

2 cups loosely packed fresh flat-leaf parsley, roughly chopped

1 cup sliced green onion tops

1 cup loosely packed fresh dill, roughly chopped

1 cup canned chickpeas, rinsed and drained

¼ cup lemon juice (from 1½ to 2 lemons)

¼ cup extra-virgin olive oil

1 teaspoon dried oregano

½ cup raw pine nuts

Salt and freshly ground black pepper to taste

Optional: Add crumbled sheep's milk feta cheese to the salad for a vegetarian version.

1. Heat 2 cups water and the quinoa in a medium pot over high heat until the water boils. Reduce the heat to low, cover the pot, and cook for 15 minutes, or until the quinoa has absorbed all the water.

2. While the quinoa is cooking, combine the cucumber, tomatoes, parsley, green onions, dill, and chickpeas in a large bowl.

recipe continues

3. Combine the lemon juice, olive oil, and oregano in a mason jar. Cover and shake well to combine the ingredients.

4. Pour the dressing over the quinoa and vegetables. Add the pine nuts and stir well to combine all the ingredients. Season with salt and pepper.

Pro Tip

Swap the chickpeas for rinsed and drained canned lentils or cannellini beans. Use any variety of fresh herbs, including mint, cilantro, and basil. Store the quinoa salad in a well-sealed container in the refrigerator for up to 4 days.

Creamy Miso-Peanut Noodle Bowl

13 PLANT POINTS

Craving a quick, protein-packed meal? These creamy miso-peanut noodles with broccoli, carrots, and tofu bring plenty of flavor thanks to a savory-sweet sauce of peanut butter, miso, and tamari. This nourishing pasta dish will become a new favorite on your dinner rotation menu!

SERVES 4

TOTAL TIME: 30 MINUTES (20 MINUTES ACTIVE TIME)

One 8-ounce package of chickpea linguine noodles

15 ounces firm tofu (organic), drained

½ cup natural peanut butter

¼ cup apple cider vinegar

1 tablespoon low-sodium gluten-free tamari

1 tablespoon gluten-free miso

1 teaspoon garlic-infused oil

2 teaspoons 100% maple syrup

1 tablespoon extra-virgin olive oil

3 cups bite-sized broccoli crown florets

2 cups shredded carrots

Salt and freshly ground black pepper to taste

1 cup fresh cilantro, roughly chopped

1 cup sliced green onion tops

1 cup mung bean sprouts

½ cup raw peanuts, roughly chopped

2 limes, cut into quarters

Red pepper flakes to taste (optional)

Optional: Top with Easy Pan-Seared Salmon (page 366) for a pescatarian version.

1. Bring a large pot of water to a boil over high heat. Add the pasta and cook according to the package directions and desired doneness. Stir it regularly to keep the noodles from sticking together.

recipe continues

2. Slice the tofu into ½-inch cubes and set aside in a small bowl.

3. Make the sauce while the pasta is cooking: Combine the peanut butter, vinegar, tamari, miso, garlic oil, and maple syrup in a bowl. Add water to thin slightly to the desired consistency.

4. Heat a large skillet over medium heat. Add the olive oil to the pan and then the broccoli. Sauté for 3 minutes. Add the carrots and sauté for 2 minutes. Season with salt and pepper.

5. Drain the pasta once cooked, then add it to the pan with the vegetables. Stir in the cubed tofu and sauce and toss well to combine the ingredients.

6. To serve: Divide the pasta among 4 bowls. Top each bowl with cilantro, green onions, mung bean sprouts, and peanuts. Serve with lime wedges and red pepper flakes, if desired.

Garden Green Spud Salad

9 PLANT POINTS

Calling all potato lovers! This Garden Green Spud Salad is a potato lover's dream with Indian-inspired herbs and spices! This recipe is even better as leftovers. When we cook then cool our potatoes, we increase the resistant starch in them to feed our gut bugs.

SERVES 6

TOTAL TIME: 50 MINUTES (20 MINUTES ACTIVE TIME)

2 pounds red potatoes, cut into ½-inch cubes

4 cups loosely packed fresh cilantro, leaves and stems

2 cups loosely packed fresh mint

1 tablespoon garlic-infused oil

6 tablespoons extra-virgin olive oil

½ cup almond milk yogurt

½ teaspoon ground cumin

1 lime, juiced

½ teaspoon salt or to taste

Freshly ground black pepper to taste

Sliced jalapeño to taste (optional)

One 15-ounce can lentils, rinsed and drained (1½ cups)

1 cup sliced green onion tops

Optional: Pescatarians will love this with Easy Pan-Seared Salmon (page 366) for a tasty anti-inflammatory meal! Craving more greens? Serve on top of a bed of baby arugula. Want a little crunch? Top with pumpkin seeds.

1. Place the potatoes in a medium to large pot and cover with water, 2 inches above the potatoes. Bring to a boil over high heat, then reduce the heat to low and simmer for 10 minutes, or until the potatoes are tender. Drain the potatoes, transfer to a bowl, and place in the refrigerator to cool for 30 minutes.

recipe continues

2. Prepare the sauce while the potatoes are cooking and cooling: Combine the cilantro, mint, garlic oil, olive oil, yogurt, cumin, lime juice, salt, pepper, and jalapeño, if using, in a blender. Blend on high speed until smooth and creamy.

3. When the potatoes are cool, add the lentils to the bowl, along with the green sauce. Stir well to combine and season with additional salt and pepper if desired.

4. Divide among 6 serving bowls and top each serving with the green onions.

Pro Tip

White potatoes can be used in place of red potatoes. Swap the almond milk yogurt with lactose-free yogurt for a vegetarian version. Store the salad in a sealed container in the refrigerator for up to 4 days.

Sweet Potato Lentil Curry

11 PLANT POINTS

This nourishing Sweet Potato Lentil Curry is a cozy meal to warm up your insides. Packed with protein and fiber, this flavorful curry is gentle on your digestive tract. Serve it over a brown rice or quinoa bed for a comforting and satisfying lunch or dinner.

SERVES 4
TOTAL TIME: 35 MINUTES (20 MINUTES ACTIVE TIME)

1 tablespoon extra-virgin olive oil

1 cup sliced leeks, green tops only

1 cup canned lentils, rinsed and drained

One 10-ounce bag of frozen sweet potato chunks (no need to thaw)

2 teaspoons grated fresh ginger

1 teaspoon curry powder

½ teaspoon garam masala

1 cup canned crushed or diced tomatoes in juice

1 cup P3 Biome Broth (page 285) or water

½ cup light coconut milk

¾ teaspoon salt or to taste

Freshly ground black pepper to taste

3 cups frozen or precooked brown rice, for serving

½ cup lightly packed fresh cilantro, chopped

Optional: Serve with a dollop of yogurt (almond or lactose-free plain unsweetened yogurt) on top or add a small portion of Stovetop Shrimp (page 367). Want some crunch? Top with slivered almonds.

1. Heat the olive oil in a medium or large pot over medium-high heat. Add the leeks and sauté for 2 minutes, or until softened.

recipe continues

2. Add the lentils, sweet potatoes, ginger, curry powder, garam masala, tomatoes, broth, and coconut milk. Bring to a boil, reduce the heat to low, and simmer for 15 minutes.

3. Season with the salt and pepper.

4. Divide the rice among 4 serving bowls and top with the curry and cilantro.

Pro Tip

Prepare this curry ahead of time and store it in a well-sealed container in the refrigerator for 3 to 4 days or in the freezer for 3 to 4 months.

Wild Rice Power Bowl

9 PLANT POINTS

Experience the hearty, nutty flavor of wild rice in this power bowl enhanced by sweet potatoes, green beans, and toasty hazelnuts. Prep it for dinner and then enjoy the leftovers another day for lunch.

SERVES 2
TOTAL TIME: 50 MINUTES (25 MINUTES ACTIVE TIME)

½ cup wild rice, well rinsed

¼ cup plus 1 tablespoon extra-virgin olive oil

¼ cup freshly squeezed orange juice (about 1 orange)

½ teaspoon Dijon mustard

Salt and freshly ground black pepper to taste

½ cup raw hazelnuts

1 cup frozen sweet potato chunks

1½ cups frozen green beans

½ cup fresh tarragon, roughly chopped

½ cup fresh flat-leaf parsley, roughly chopped

Optional: If desired, add a soft-boiled egg (page 365) or a piece of Easy Pan-Seared Salmon (page 366).

1. Add the rinsed wild rice and 1¼ cups water to a small or medium pot. Bring to a boil over high heat, then reduce the heat to low, cover the pot, and cook for 45 minutes. After the rice is cooked and the water has evaporated, remove the pot from the heat and allow it to steam with the cover on for 10 minutes.

2. While the rice is cooking, prepare the dressing and the other ingredients: Combine ¼ cup of the olive oil, the orange juice,

recipe continues

mustard, and salt and pepper in a mixing bowl or small mason jar. Stir well or cover and shake to combine the ingredients.

3. Heat the hazelnuts over medium-high heat in a skillet. Stir constantly for 4 minutes. Remove from the heat immediately and allow the nuts to cool for 5 minutes. Lightly chop the hazelnuts and set aside.

4. Combine the frozen sweet potatoes and green beans in a microwave-safe bowl with 2 tablespoons water. Heat the vegetables in the microwave for 3½ minutes, or until cooked. Drain the water from the vegetables, return to the bowl, and toss with the remaining 1 tablespoon olive oil and salt and pepper to taste.

5. Divide the rice between 2 serving bowls. Top each bowl with half of the vegetables and half of the nuts. Drizzle the dressing on top of each bowl (you may have extra) and garnish each serving with tarragon and parsley.

Pro Tip

Prep all of the ingredients (rice, vegetables, and nuts) and store them in individual sealed containers for 3 to 4 days. The rice and vegetables should be stored in the refrigerator.

Edamame Guacamole

7 PLANT POINTS

Eating such a small amount of avocado on the low FODMAP diet can be challenging. Enter edamame beans to the rescue! Complete the guacamole recipe with flavorful cilantro, green onions, garlic oil, and jalapeño for a tasty high-protein dip.

SERVES 4
TOTAL TIME: 10 MINUTES

2 cups frozen shelled edamame, thawed

1 medium avocado, peeled

1 cup loosely packed fresh cilantro

½ cup sliced green onion tops

1 medium lime, juiced (about 2 tablespoons)

2 tablespoons extra-virgin olive oil

2 teaspoons garlic-infused oil

Salt and freshly ground black pepper to taste

1 jalapeño (optional)

1. Add the edamame, avocado, cilantro, green onions, lime juice, olive oil, and garlic oil to the bowl of a food processor. Process until smooth and creamy, scraping down the bowl as needed.

2. Add salt, pepper, and jalapeño to taste, if using, and process to mix the ingredients.

Pro Tip

Spread guacamole on sourdough toast and top with sliced tomato and any fresh herbs. Or serve with low FODMAP crackers.

Citrus and Herb Toasted Nut Mix

6 PLANT POINTS

Want a super-easy, healthy, nourishing snack? Grab a handful of nuts and nosh away. Take your nuts to the next level with EVOO, rosemary, and lemon zest. Absolutely divine!

SERVES 8
TOTAL TIME: 10 MINUTES

1 tablespoon extra-virgin olive oil

2 tablespoons finely chopped fresh rosemary

1 small lemon, zested

¼ teaspoon salt or to taste

Freshly ground black pepper to taste

¾ cup raw pecans, roughly chopped

¾ cup raw walnuts, roughly chopped

½ cup raw Brazil nuts, roughly chopped

1. Combine the olive oil, rosemary, lemon zest, salt, and pepper in a medium bowl. Stir well to combine.

2. Add the nuts to the olive oil mixture and toss to coat.

3. Heat a medium to large skillet over medium heat. Add the nuts and sauté for 4 minutes, or until lightly toasted. Remove from the skillet immediately to stop the cooking.

4. Allow the nuts to cool before serving.

5. Store the nuts in a well-sealed container for up to 1 week.

Pro Tip
Feel free to use any variety of low FODMAP nuts—peanuts, pine nuts, hazelnuts, and macadamia nuts—in addition to the above.

5-Ingredient Energy Bites

5 PLANT POINTS

When you want something sweet, these double-nut energy bites will satisfy all your cravings. Make a big batch to store in the freezer for up to 1 month. They're low in sugar but packed with nutrition and yummy for your tummy!

SERVES 12
TOTAL TIME: 10 MINUTES

---

1 cup raw walnuts

1 cup raw pecans

3 tablespoons ground flaxseed

1 tablespoon plus 1 teaspoon 100% maple syrup or to taste

1 teaspoon vanilla extract

⅛ teaspoon salt or to taste

1. Add the walnuts and pecans to the bowl of a food processor and process for 45 seconds, or until the nut mixture pulls away from the bowl's sides.

2. Add the flaxseed, maple syrup, vanilla, and salt and pulse for 15 to 30 seconds, until the ingredients are well combined.

3. Shape the mixture into about 12 bites/balls. If the mixture seems too dry for shaping, you might add a teaspoon or two of water (or extra maple syrup) so it sticks together.

4. Store in an airtight container in the refrigerator for up to 1 week or in the freezer for up to 1 month.

Chocolate Raspberry Chia Parfait

6 PLANT POINTS

Chocolate and berries are the perfect polyphenol-rich pairing! This delicious parfait combines chocolate yogurt with chia seeds and raspberries for a satisfying high-fiber snack or dessert.

SERVES 2

TOTAL TIME: 30 MINUTES (5 MINUTES ACTIVE TIME)

---

1 cup almond milk yogurt

2 tablespoons unsweetened cocoa powder

2 tablespoons chia seeds

1 tablespoon 100% maple syrup

½ teaspoon vanilla extract

⅔ cup frozen raspberries, thawed

2 teaspoons dark chocolate (at least 70% cacao) chips

Optional: Lactose-free plain unsweetened yogurt can be used in place of the almond milk yogurt if desired.

1. Combine the yogurt, cocoa powder, chia seeds, maple syrup, and vanilla in a mixing bowl. Stir well to combine the ingredients.

2. Divide the chia seed mixture into 2 small serving bowls and refrigerate for 30 minutes to thicken. If you prefer a thicker texture, you might stir the mixture once or twice during the 30-minute chill to ensure that the chia seeds are evenly distributed.

3. To serve: Divide the raspberries and chocolate chips between the bowls.

4. Store in the refrigerator for up to 4 days.

Pro Tip

You can swap the raspberries for blueberries or strawberries (stick to 10 strawberries total, or 5 per serving, to keep it low FODMAP).

Summer Garden Blended Juice

7 PLANT POINTS

Refresh and revitalize with this hydrating, nutrient-packed drink that tastes like summer in a glass.

SERVES 3
TOTAL TIME: 7 MINUTES

3 medium tomatoes (heirloom if available), roughly chopped

½ red bell pepper, roughly chopped

½ cucumber, peeled and roughly chopped (about ¾ cup)

½ cup sliced green onion tops

½ cup roughly chopped fresh flat-leaf parsley

½ cup roughly chopped fresh cilantro

1 lemon, juiced

Jalapeño to taste (optional)

Salt and freshly ground black pepper to taste (optional)

1. Add the tomatoes, bell pepper, cucumber, green onion, parsley, cilantro, and lemon juice to a blender. Blend on high speed until the ingredients are well combined.

2. Season with jalapeño, salt, and pepper if desired, blending to combine all of the ingredients.

3. Serve over ice.

4. Store the juice in the refrigerator in a well-sealed container for up to 4 days. Shake well before serving.

Top Secret Mango Lassi

4 PLANT POINTS

Satisfy your craving for tropical sweetness with this Top Secret Mango Lassi—complete with a fiber-boosting secret ingredient: lentils! Shhh . . . Don't tell anyone. It's our secret.

SERVES 1
TOTAL TIME: 5 MINUTES

½ cup almond milk, or more for a thinner consistency if desired

½ cup almond milk yogurt

1 cup frozen mango

½ cup canned lentils, rinsed and drained

½ teaspoon ground ginger

100% maple syrup for added sweetness (optional)

Pinch of salt (optional)

Optional: Use lactose-free plain unsweetened yogurt instead of almond milk yogurt for additional protein. Garnish with slivered almonds for a little crunch.

1. Add the almond milk, yogurt, mango, lentils, and ginger to a blender. Blend on high speed until smooth.

2. Add maple syrup to taste and a pinch of salt, if desired, and blend again.

3. Pour into a glass and serve.

Spiced Pomegranate Lassi

7 PLANT POINTS

Enjoy a sweet-tart burst of pomegranate, balanced by a swirl of creamy yogurt and warming spices in this Spiced Pomegranate Lassi. Each sip delivers a dose of polyphenols and gut-friendly probiotics for a vibrant, refreshing treat any time of day.

SERVES 1
TOTAL TIME: 10 MINUTES

¾ cup pomegranate arils, frozen or fresh, plus more for garnish

½ cup almond milk

½ cup almond milk yogurt

½ lemon, juiced

2 teaspoons 100% maple syrup

¼ teaspoon ground cinnamon

⅛ teaspoon ground cardamom

⅛ teaspoon ground ginger

Pinch of salt (optional)

1 teaspoon raw pine nuts, for garnish (optional)

Ice, for serving

Optional: Use lactose-free plain unsweetened yogurt instead of almond milk yogurt if desired.

1. Combine the pomegranate arils, almond milk, yogurt, lemon juice, maple syrup, cinnamon, cardamom, ginger, and salt, if desired, in a blender. Blend on high speed until smooth. If you like a smoother texture and you're using fresh pomegranate arils, you may wish to strain the smoothie after blending to remove any leftover seed bits.

2. Pour over ice, garnish with extra pomegranate arils and pine nuts, if desired, and serve.

15-Minute Tortilla Soup

6 PLANT POINTS

Make this nourishing and delicious tortilla soup in 15 minutes! Make a big batch ahead of time to freeze and enjoy it with your favorite toppings.

SERVES 4
TOTAL TIME: 15 MINUTES

---

4 cups P3 Biome Broth (page 285) or water

One 14.5-ounce can diced tomatoes

One 15-ounce can black bean, rinsed and drained

1½ cups frozen corn

1½ teaspoons ground cumin or to taste

2 teaspoons chili powder or to taste

Salt and freshly ground black pepper to taste

4 corn tortillas

1 tablespoon extra-virgin olive oil

Optional: Add avocado, radishes, pumpkin seeds, and/or chopped cilantro.

1. Preheat the oven to 400°F. Line a baking sheet with parchment paper.

2. While the oven is preheating, combine the broth, tomatoes, beans, corn, cumin, chili powder, salt, and pepper in a medium to large pot. Bring to a boil over high heat, then reduce the temperature and simmer while the chips are baking.

3. Brush one side of each tortilla with olive oil, then cut into strips. Lay the tortilla strips on the parchment-lined baking

recipe continues

sheet and bake for 7 minutes, or until they have reached the desired level of crispness. Remove the chips from the oven.

4. While the tortilla chips are baking, prep the optional toppings, if using, and place them in bowls.

5. To serve: Divide the chips into 4 serving bowls and ladle soup on top. Let everyone add their toppings as desired.

6. Store the soup in an airtight container in the refrigerator for up to 4 days or in the freezer (allow room in the container for expansion) for up to 6 months.

Pre and Pro Miso Bowl

4 PLANT POINTS

A swirl of miso paste lends subtle richness and beneficial probiotics, while sweet corn and fresh green onions bring color and crunch. Ready in minutes, this is an easy, nourishing meal you can customize with your favorite low FODMAP vegetables.

SERVES 2

TOTAL TIME: 20 MINUTES (10 MINUTES ACTIVE TIME)

---

1 large carrot, diced (about 1 cup)

4 cups P3 Biome Broth (page 285) or water

4 tablespoons miso (e.g., mellow white miso; read labels if certified gluten-free miso is preferred)

½ cup frozen corn

7½ ounces firm tofu (organic), cut into cubes (about 1¾ cups)

½ cup sliced green onion tops

Optional: Add in additional low FODMAP vegetables as desired. Suggestions include bok choy, bamboo shoots, cabbage, green beans, and low FODMAP leafy greens.

1. Combine the carrot and broth in a medium pot and bring to a boil over high heat.

2. Whisk the miso in a small amount of hot water before adding it to the soup, to allow it to blend better.

3. Add the corn and tofu and simmer for 5 minutes.

4. Divide into 2 bowls and top each bowl with green onions.

recipe continues

5. Store the soup in an airtight container in the refrigerator for up to 4 days or in the freezer (allow room in the container for expansion) for up to 6 months.

Pro Tip

To preserve the probiotic benefits of miso, avoid boiling it. Reduce the heat to low and add the miso, keeping the soup at a gentle simmer, not a full boil.

Peanut Pumpkin Power Bowl

7 PLANT POINTS

Rich peanut butter and sweet pumpkin puree swirl together atop hearty chia-infused oats in this quick, protein-packed breakfast bowl. Best of all, it's ready in minutes—ideal for busy mornings.

SERVES 1

TOTAL TIME: 10 MINUTES (5 MINUTES ACTIVE TIME)

¼ cup gluten-free oats (organic)

2 tablespoons chia seeds

½ cup almond milk

2 teaspoons 100% maple syrup

⅛ teaspoon salt (optional)

1 tablespoon natural peanut butter

1 tablespoon canned pumpkin puree

1 tablespoon chopped raw pecans

1 tablespoon pumpkin seeds

1. Combine the oats, chia seeds, almond milk, 1 teaspoon of the maple syrup, and the salt, if using, in a microwave-safe bowl. Heat in the microwave for 1 minute. Stir, then heat for an additional minute. Remove from the microwave and let the oatmeal rest for 5 minutes to thicken further.

2. Combine the peanut butter, pumpkin, and the remaining teaspoon of maple syrup in a small microwave-safe bowl. Heat for approximately 20 seconds, or until the mixture is slightly melted. Stir the peanut-pumpkin mixture into the oatmeal.

3. To serve: Top with the pecans and pumpkin seeds.

4. Store leftover pumpkin puree in an airtight container in the refrigerator for up to 4 days or in the freezer for up to 4 months.

Cherry Pie Chia Pudding

5 PLANT POINTS

This Cherry Pie Chia Pudding layers fiber-rich chia seeds and tangy-sweet cherries in a silky almond milk base for a guilt-free indulgence.

SERVES 3
TOTAL TIME: 40 MINUTES (10 MINUTES ACTIVE TIME)

1½ cups almond milk

1 tablespoon 100% maple syrup or to taste

2 teaspoons vanilla extract

½ cup chia seeds

Pinch of salt (optional)

1½ cups frozen cherries, thawed

3 tablespoons sliced or slivered raw almonds

Optional: You can substitute lactose-free plain unsweetened yogurt for almond yogurt if desired.

1. Combine the almond milk, maple syrup, vanilla, chia seeds, and salt, if using, in a mixing bowl or large mason jar. Stir or cover and shake well to combine the ingredients. Let rest for 5 minutes, then stir or shake again. Repeat after another 5 minutes, then place the mixture in the refrigerator for 20 minutes, or until thickened. Alternatively, you can let it chill longer (even overnight) for an even thicker texture.

2. To serve: Layer half of the chia pudding into 3 serving dishes. Top each serving with ¼ cup of the cherries and 1½ teaspoons of the almonds. Repeat with the remaining chia pudding, cherries, and almonds.

3. Store the chia pudding in the refrigerator for up to 4 days.

Speedy Chickpea Shakshuka

9 PLANT POINTS

Craving a hearty one-pan meal in minutes? This Speedy Chickpea Shakshuka swaps eggs for protein-packed tofu and chickpeas, all simmered in a fragrant tomato sauce. It's delicious on its own or served with a few slices of your favorite sourdough toast—perfect for soaking up every last drop.

SERVES 4
TOTAL TIME: 15 MINUTES

---

1 tablespoon extra-virgin olive oil

1 tablespoon garlic-infused oil

1 cup sliced leeks, green part only

One 15-ounce can chickpeas, rinsed and drained

2 teaspoons smoked paprika

1 teaspoon fennel seeds

1 teaspoon salt or to taste

Freshly ground black pepper to taste

One 28-ounce can crushed tomatoes

12 ounces firm tofu (organic), cut into cubes

Sourdough bread, for serving (optional)

Optional: If you want a more traditional shakshuka style, crack a few eggs into the simmering sauce. Garnish with flat-leaf parsley or microgreens.

1. Heat the olive oil and garlic oil in a medium or large skillet over medium-high heat. Add the leeks and sauté for 3 minutes, or until softened.

2. Add the chickpeas, paprika, fennel seeds, salt, and pepper to the skillet. Sauté for 1 minute.

recipe continues

3. Add the crushed tomatoes and tofu to the skillet. Reduce the heat to low and simmer for 10 minutes.

4. Divide into 4 bowls and serve with the optional bread.

5. Store the shakshuka in a well-sealed container in the refrigerator for up to 4 days or in the freezer (allow room in the container for expansion) for up to 1 month.

Avocado Toast with a Dukkah Twist

7 PLANT POINTS

Ready to elevate your avocado toast game? This version sprinkles on homemade dukkah—a fragrant Middle Eastern blend of pecans, seeds, and warm spices. The result is a nutrient-dense delight you'll crave at breakfast, lunch, or whenever hunger strikes.

SERVES 1
TOTAL TIME: 10 MINUTES

Dukkah

½ cup raw pecans

2 tablespoons sesame seeds

1 teaspoon fennel seeds

½ teaspoon ground coriander

½ teaspoon ground cumin

⅛ teaspoon salt or to taste

Avocado Toast

2 slices sourdough bread

½ avocado, peeled and sliced

Tomato slices (optional)

Optional: Add smoked salmon or a soft-boiled egg (page 365) to the avocado toast if desired.

1. Make the dukkah: Add the pecans, sesame seeds, fennel seeds, coriander, cumin, and salt to the bowl of a mini food processor. Process until finely chopped, being careful not to overprocess the mixture into a paste.

2. Make the toast: Toast the bread and top each slice with avocado slices, tomato slices, if desired, and 1 tablespoon of the dukkah seasoning.

Pro Tip

Make the dukkah ahead of time and store it in an airtight container in the refrigerator for up to 2 weeks. Having this flavorful seasoning on hand is a game changer—sprinkle it generously over soups, salads, grain bowls, or roasted veggies to instantly transform everyday dishes into gourmet creations. Chef's kiss!

Morning Sundae Surprise

5 PLANT POINTS

This high-protein "sundae" sneaks in lentils for an extra fiber and protein boost, while frozen banana and peanut butter create a luscious ice cream–like texture.

SERVES 1
TOTAL TIME: 5 MINUTES

1 frozen ripe banana, sliced

½ cup canned, rinsed, and drained lentils, optionally frozen (see note)

¼ cup almond milk, plus more as needed

1 tablespoon natural peanut butter

1 tablespoon unsweetened cocoa powder

2 tablespoons salted peanuts

2 teaspoons cacao nibs

Optional: Almond yogurt or lactose-free plain unsweetened yogurt can be added as a topping if desired.

1. Combine the banana, lentils, almond milk, peanut butter, and cocoa powder in a high-powered blender. Blend on high, using a tamper device, and periodically scrape the sides of the blender as needed until all of the ingredients are well combined and the mixture has a creamy consistency. If the mixture seems too thick, add a splash more almond milk.

2. Spoon the mixture into a serving glass or bowl and top with peanuts and cacao nibs.

Pro Tip

Frozen lentils give the sundae an ice cream/milkshake consistency. To make frozen lentils, lay the cooked lentils on a parchment paper–lined baking sheet. Pat the lentils dry to remove any excess liquid. Place the baking sheet in the freezer. Once the lentils are fully frozen, store them in a well-sealed bag in the freezer for up to 1 month.

Crunchy Tempeh Tacos

10 PLANT POINTS

Tempeh is a tasty fermented soy protein that's also a source of probiotics. Its tangy flavor pairs well with warm spices like chili powder and cumin. Sauté it in a skillet like ground meat, and pair it with homemade guacamole and a spread of veggie toppings for a wonderful taco night any day of the week.

SERVES 3
TOTAL TIME: 20 MINUTES

---

2 tablespoons avocado oil

8 ounces tempeh, crumbled

2 teaspoons chili powder

1 teaspoon dried oregano

½ teaspoon ground cumin

¾ teaspoon salt or to taste

Freshly ground black pepper to taste

6 corn hard taco shells

2 medium avocados, peeled

½ lime, juiced

½ cup chopped fresh cilantro

1 teaspoon garlic-infused oil

Finely chopped jalapeño to taste (optional)

½ cup sliced green onion tops

Optional: Add chopped romaine lettuce, tomatoes, almond milk yogurt, or lactose-free plain unsweetened yogurt.

1. Preheat the oven to 325°F.

2. Heat the avocado oil in a medium skillet over medium-high heat. Add the tempeh and sauté for 2 minutes.

3. Add the chili powder, oregano, cumin, 2 to 3 tablespoons water, the salt, and pepper. Sauté for 2 minutes, then remove from the heat while you prepare the other ingredients.

4. Place the taco shells on a baking pan and bake for 5 minutes.

5. Prepare the guacamole while the taco shells are baking. In a medium bowl, combine the avocados, lime juice, ¼ cup of the cilantro, the garlic oil, and salt and pepper. Mash the avocados with a potato masher or fork and stir the ingredients to combine. Add jalapeño if desired.

6. To serve: Divide the tempeh taco mixture among the 6 tacos. Top with guacamole, the remaining ¼ cup cilantro, and green onions. Add optional toppings, including lettuce, tomato, and yogurt if desired.

Pro Tip
Make the tempeh filling ahead of time and store it in an airtight container in the refrigerator for up to 4 days.

Southwest Quinoa Salad with Cumin Lime Dressing

14 PLANT POINTS

Looking to bring some color and flavor to your table? This Southwest Quinoa Salad with Cumin Lime Dressing does the trick. Make it ahead and enjoy it for several meals throughout the week.

SERVES 6
TOTAL TIME: 25 MINUTES

1½ cups quinoa, rinsed

¼ cup lime juice (about 3 limes)

½ cup extra-virgin olive oil

¼ cup white balsamic vinegar

½ teaspoon dried oregano

½ teaspoon ground cumin

¼ teaspoon salt or to taste

⅛ teaspoon freshly ground black pepper or to taste

One 15-ounce can black beans, rinsed and drained

1 cup frozen corn

1 medium orange bell pepper, diced (about 1½ cups)

1 cup loosely packed fresh cilantro, chopped

½ cup sliced radishes

¾ cup sliced green onion tops

1 cup sliced cherry or grape tomatoes

Optional: Add Stovetop Shrimp (page 367) if desired. Pumpkin seeds or sunflower seeds add a nice crunch.

1. Cook the quinoa according to the package directions. Fluff with a fork when finished cooking.

2. While the quinoa is cooking, make the dressing: Combine the lime juice, olive oil, vinegar, oregano, cumin, salt, and pepper in a large mason jar. Cover and shake well to combine the ingredients.

3. Add the cooked quinoa to a large bowl with the beans, corn, bell pepper, cilantro, radishes, green onion, and tomatoes.

4. Pour the dressing on top of the salad and stir well to combine. Season to taste with additional salt and pepper if desired.

Pro Tip
Make the salad ahead of time and store it in a well-sealed container in the refrigerator for up to 4 days.

Citrus Kale Pasta Salad

8 PLANT POINTS

Despite the simple ingredients list, this Citrus Kale Pasta Salad is full of fiber and flavor. It's perfect for a quick lunch or light dinner.

SERVES 4
TOTAL TIME: 15 MINUTES

---

8 ounces dried chickpea pasta

6 tablespoons extra-virgin olive oil

1 teaspoon garlic-infused oil

¼ cup lemon juice

4 cups chopped kale

1 cup raw pistachios, chopped

Salt, freshly ground black pepper, and crushed red pepper flakes to taste

Optional: Add Stovetop Shrimp (page 367) if desired and use organic whole-wheat pasta if you have no gluten concerns. Sheep's milk feta cheese or goat cheese provides extra protein and flavor for a vegetarian version.

1. Cook the pasta according to the package directions, then drain and transfer to a large bowl.

2. Make the dressing: Combine the olive oil, garlic oil, and lemon juice in a jar and shake well.

3. To the bowl with the pasta, add the kale and pistachios. Pour the dressing on top and toss well. Season with salt, pepper, and red pepper flakes.

4. Serve warm or at room temperature.

Pro Tip

Make the pasta salad ahead of time and store it in a well-sealed container in the refrigerator for up to 4 days. Gluten-free pasta can get dried out in the refrigerator. If this happens, briefly reheat the pasta salad in the microwave before serving.

Double Strawberry Spring Salad

6 PLANT POINTS

This dreamy salad packs a double strawberry punch, featuring strawberries in the dressing and on top of the salad. Arugula serves as a base, and slivered almonds give it a delicious crunch. Serve it as a side salad or topped with your favorite protein.

SERVES 2
TOTAL TIME: 10 MINUTES

2 tablespoons extra-virgin olive oil

1 tablespoon lemon juice

1 tablespoon white balsamic vinegar

5 whole strawberries, hulled, plus 2 cups sliced strawberries

Salt and freshly ground black pepper to taste

6 cups baby arugula

½ cup slivered raw almonds

Optional: Enjoy with Crispy Baked Tofu (page 362), The *Best* Tempeh (page 363), or Easy Pan-Seared Salmon (page 366) for a complete meal. Add microgreens or sprouts as desired.

1. Combine the olive oil, lemon juice, vinegar, the 5 whole strawberries, and salt and pepper in a blender. Blend on high speed until smooth and creamy.

2. Assemble the salads: Divide the arugula between 2 plates. Top each with sliced strawberries, almonds, and optional ingredients, if using. Drizzle the dressing over the salad.

Spiced Chickpea and Beet Yogurt Bowl

10 PLANT POINTS

This Middle Eastern–inspired creation layers creamy yogurt with crispy spiced chickpeas, sweet earthy beets, and peppery arugula. The result is a beautifully balanced meal brimming with fiber, protein, and probiotics—perfect for a nourishing lunch or light dinner.

SERVES 1
TOTAL TIME: 15 MINUTES

Spiced Chickpeas

1 teaspoon smoked paprika

¾ teaspoon ground cumin

½ teaspoon ground coriander

½ teaspoon ground turmeric

½ teaspoon salt or to taste

2 tablespoons extra-virgin olive oil

One 15-ounce can chickpeas, rinsed and drained

Yogurt Bowl

⅔ cup almond milk yogurt

1 cup baby arugula

½ cup diced cooked beets

½ cup Spiced Chickpeas

½ lemon

Optional: Substitute a plain unsweetened lactose-free yogurt for a vegetarian version.

1. Make the chickpeas: Combine the paprika, cumin, coriander, turmeric, and salt in a small bowl and stir well to combine. Heat the olive oil in a medium skillet over medium-high heat. Add the chickpeas and spices and stir well to combine. Cook, stirring occasionally, for 8 minutes, or until the chickpeas get crispy.

recipe continues

2. Assemble the bowl: Add the yogurt to a serving bowl, along with the arugula, beets, and chickpeas. Serve with lemon wedges.

Pro Tip

Make the spiced chickpeas ahead of time and store them in an airtight container in the refrigerator for up to 4 days.

Springtime Panzanella Salad

9 PLANT POINTS

If you've never had panzanella salad, you're in for a big treat! This Tuscan-inspired salad combines toasted bread with asparagus, greens, and beans for the ultimate healthy comfort meal!

SERVES 3
TOTAL TIME: 20 MINUTES

4 slices sourdough bread (gluten-free if desired)

4 tablespoons extra-virgin olive oil, plus more for the bread

Salt and freshly ground black pepper to taste

2 tablespoons lemon juice

1 tablespoon white balsamic vinegar

1 cup sliced asparagus (1-inch pieces)

2 cups baby arugula

One 15-ounce can cannellini beans, rinsed and drained

½ cup chopped fresh mint

¼ cup torn fresh tarragon

Optional: Substitute gluten-free bread if desired. Consider Stovetop Shrimp (page 367), Crispy Baked Tofu (page 362), or The *Best* Tempeh (page 363) for extra protein if desired.

1. Preheat the oven to 400°F. Line a baking sheet with aluminum foil.

2. Cut the bread into 1-inch cubes. Place it on the foil-lined baking sheet, drizzle with olive oil, season with pepper, and toss with your hands to coat all the cubes. Bake for 5 minutes, or until lightly browned. Remove from the oven and set aside while you make the rest of the salad.

recipe continues

3. Make the dressing: Combine 3 tablespoons of the olive oil, the lemon juice, and vinegar in a mason jar. Season with salt and pepper. Cover and shake well to combine the ingredients.

4. Heat a medium skillet over medium-high heat. Add the remaining 1 tablespoon of olive oil to the skillet along with the asparagus. Sauté for 5 minutes, or until the asparagus is tender.

5. Add the arugula to a large serving bowl along with the cooked asparagus, beans, toasted bread cubes, mint, and tarragon. Top with the salad dressing and toss well to combine. Season with additional salt and pepper if desired.

Mulligatawny Soup

11 PLANT POINTS

This sweet and savory Anglo-Indian soup is a flavorful concoction of apples, rice, vegetables, and warming spices. Some versions add chicken, but this plant-based recipe features lentils for protein. Make a big batch, as you'll be sure to want leftovers!

SERVES 4
TOTAL TIME: 45 MINUTES (30 MINUTES ACTIVE TIME)

3 tablespoons extra-virgin olive oil

1 stalk celery, chopped

1½ cups sliced leeks, green tops only

1 cup chopped carrot

4 teaspoons curry powder

1 tablespoon chopped fresh thyme, or 1 teaspoon dried

1 teaspoon ground cinnamon

1 teaspoon salt or to taste

Freshly ground black pepper to taste

4 cups P3 Biome Broth (page 285) or water

2 cups finely diced peeled Honeycrisp or other sweet-tart apple (about 1½ apples)

2 cups frozen precooked brown rice

1 cup canned lentils, rinsed and drained

½ cup light coconut milk

Almond milk yogurt, for serving (optional)

Chopped fresh cilantro, for serving (optional)

Optional: Stir in cooked chickpeas or tofu cubes for extra plant-based protein. Lactose-free plain unsweetened yogurt can be used in place of the almond milk yogurt for a vegetarian version.

recipe continues

1. Heat a medium to large stockpot over medium-high heat. Add the olive oil, celery, leeks, and carrots and sauté for 5 minutes.

2. Add the curry powder, thyme, cinnamon, salt, and pepper to the vegetables and stir well to combine.

3. Add the broth, apples, rice, and lentils. Bring the ingredients to a boil, reduce the heat to low, cover the pot, and simmer for 10 minutes.

4. Remove the pot from the heat and use an immersion blender to slightly puree the ingredients. Keep the soup a little chunky for the best texture.

5. Stir in the coconut milk, divide into 4 bowls, and top with the yogurt and cilantro to serve, if using.

6. Store the soup in an airtight container in the refrigerator for up to 4 days or in the freezer (allow room in the container for expansion) for up to 6 months.

Eat the Rainbow Salad

15 PLANT POINTS

Brighten up your plate with this colorful salad featuring crispy baked tofu, creamy avocado, and crunchy peanuts tied together by a tangy-sweet citrus dressing.

SERVES 2

TOTAL TIME: 25 MINUTES (15 MINUTES ACTIVE TIME)

3 tablespoons avocado oil

1 tablespoon gluten-free tamari

1 tablespoon rice wine vinegar

1 teaspoon toasted sesame oil

1 teaspoon 100% maple syrup

⅛ teaspoon ground ginger

½ orange, juiced (about 2 tablespoons)

1 lime, juiced (about 1 tablespoon)

4 cups chopped romaine lettuce

¾ cup shredded carrots

¾ cup shredded purple cabbage

½ cup sliced green onion tops

½ cup roughly chopped fresh cilantro

8 ounces Crispy Baked Tofu (page 362)

1 avocado, peeled and sliced

½ cup toasted peanuts

Optional: Consider adding a sprinkle of hempseeds, edamame, or Stovetop Shrimp (page 367), if desired.

1. Make the dressing: Combine the avocado oil, tamari, rice wine vinegar, sesame oil, maple syrup, ginger, orange juice, and lime juice in a mason jar, cover, and shake well to combine the ingredients.

recipe continues

2. Add the lettuce, carrots, cabbage, green onions, and cilantro to a large bowl. Pour the dressing on top and toss to combine.

3. Divide the greens and vegetables between 2 plates. Top each plate with half the tofu, ½ avocado, and ¼ cup peanuts.

Hummus Kimchi Wraps

9 PLANT POINTS

Enjoy a flavor-packed lunch that's as simple as it is satisfying. These Hummus Kimchi Wraps feature a creamy, garlicky chickpea spread balanced by tangy kimchi and fresh arugula.

SERVES 1

TOTAL TIME: 15 MINUTES

Hummus

One 15-ounce can chickpeas, rinsed and drained

2 tablespoons extra-virgin olive oil

1 teaspoon garlic-infused oil

2 tablespoons tahini

2 tablespoons lemon juice (about ¾ lemon)

½ teaspoon ground cumin

½ teaspoon salt

Wrap

1 gluten-free low FODMAP tortilla (e.g., brown rice or corn)

⅓ cup Hummus

1 tablespoon kimchi

¾ cup baby arugula

Optional: Easy Pan-Seared Salmon (page 366) adds extra protein for pescatarians. Add thinly sliced cucumbers, bell peppers, or even a few toasted walnuts for crunch.

1. Make the hummus: Combine the chickpeas, olive oil, garlic oil, tahini, lemon juice, cumin, and salt in the bowl of a food processor. Process to blend, then scrape the sides of the bowl and process again. Add 1 tablespoon water to thin the mixture, then process again for 1 to 2 minutes, until the hummus is smooth and creamy.

recipe continues

2. Assemble the wrap: Heat the tortilla in the microwave or a skillet over medium-high heat. Spread the hummus on the tortilla and top with the kimchi and arugula. Roll into a wrap and enjoy!

3. Store the hummus in an airtight container in the refrigerator for up to 1 week. The recipe makes approximately 1½ cups of hummus so that you will have extra.

Forbidden Rice Salad

9 PLANT POINTS

Forbidden rice, also known as black rice, is an ancient variety prized for its deep purple hue and dense nutritional profile—especially its high polyphenol content. In this salad, those antioxidant-rich grains meet jewel-like pomegranate arils for a powerhouse pairing. Fresh herbs, nuts, and lentils round out the flavors in this salad, which tastes even better the next day!

SERVES 4
TOTAL TIME: 50 MINUTES (20 MINUTES ACTIVE TIME)

---

1 cup forbidden rice

2 cups pomegranate arils, fresh or frozen

1 cup canned lentils, rinsed and drained

1 cup raw walnuts, toasted and chopped

½ cup chopped fresh basil

½ cup chopped fresh mint

1 cup chopped fresh flat-leaf parsley

¼ cup extra-virgin olive oil

3 tablespoons white balsamic vinegar

¾ teaspoon salt or to taste

Freshly ground black pepper to taste

Optional: Consider adding Crispy Baked Tofu (page 362), edamame, Stovetop Shrimp (page 367), and/or Easy Pan-Seared Salmon (page 366), if desired.

1. Combine the rice and 1¾ cups water in a medium pot. Cover and bring to a boil over high heat. Reduce the heat to low and cook for 30 minutes. Remove the rice from the heat, uncover it, fluff it with a fork, and allow it to cool for 15 minutes.

recipe continues

2. While the rice is cooking, combine the pomegranate arils, lentils, walnuts, basil, mint, and parsley in a large bowl. After the rice has cooled, add it to the bowl along with the olive oil, vinegar, salt, and pepper. Stir the ingredients together to combine.

3. Divide into 4 bowls for serving.

4. Store the rice salad in the refrigerator, well covered, for up to 4 days.

Pro Tip
Substitute the walnuts for pine nuts or other nuts of choice and use any variety of fresh herbs in place of the basil, mint, and parsley.

Cashew Citrus Energy Bites

8 PLANT POINTS

Looking for a zesty pick-me-up? These Cashew Citrus Energy Bites blend cashews, oats, coconut, and bright citrus zest into sweet, chewy bites. Finished with a hempseed coating for added crunch and omega-3s, they're perfect as a quick snack or healthy dessert—enjoy with a soothing cup of matcha for ultimate snack-time bliss.

SERVES 12
TOTAL TIME: 10 MINUTES

2 cups raw cashews

¼ cup gluten-free oats (organic)

¼ cup unsweetened shredded coconut

2 tablespoons 100% maple syrup

1 teaspoon ground ginger

1 teaspoon orange zest (about ½ orange)

1 teaspoon lemon zest (about ½ lemon)

⅛ teaspoon salt or to taste

¼ cup hempseeds

1. Combine the cashews, oats, coconut, maple syrup, ginger, orange zest, lemon zest, and salt in the bowl of a food processor.

2. Process until the mixture starts to stick to the bowl. Scrape the sides and bottom of the bowl and process again until the mixture is sticky and easy to shape into balls. You may need to scrape the bowl several times to get the correct consistency.

3. Roll the mixture into about 12 equal-shaped balls.

recipe continues

4. Place the hempseeds on a plate or parchment paper and roll the balls in the hempseeds to coat.

5. Store in the refrigerator in a well-sealed container for up to 4 days or in the freezer for up to 1 month.

Chocolate-Drizzled Berry Bites

6 PLANT POINTS

Indulge your sweet tooth with these crispy rice cakes layered in peanut butter, homemade chia-raspberry jam, and a drizzle of dark chocolate. This tasty frozen concoction is a fun and healthy way to satisfy your chocolate cravings!

SERVES 5

TOTAL TIME: 30 MINUTES (15 MINUTES ACTIVE TIME)

---

1 teaspoon vegan butter

1 cup frozen raspberries

1 tablespoon chia seeds

2 teaspoons 100% maple syrup

5 rice cakes

5 tablespoons natural peanut butter

4 tablespoons dark chocolate chips (at least 70% cacao)

1. Heat a medium skillet over medium-high heat. Add the vegan butter and melt it. Add the raspberries, chia seeds, and maple syrup and cook, stirring constantly, for 4 minutes, or until the mixture thickens. Transfer the chia jam to a small bowl.

2. Line a baking sheet with parchment paper. Place the rice cakes on the sheet and spread each rice cake with 1 tablespoon peanut butter.

3. Melt the chocolate chips in the microwave on high power for 1 minute, or until melted.

recipe continues

4. Spread the chia jam, divided equally, over the rice cakes with peanut butter. Drizzle each rice cake with melted chocolate.

5. Place the sheet in the freezer for 15 minutes and serve.

6. Store the rice cakes in the freezer, in a sealed container, for up to 2 weeks.

Smoked Chili Lime Popcorn

7 PLANT POINTS

It's hard to believe something so tasty as popcorn can be a "good-for-you" fiber-rich snack, too! This easy version takes things up a notch with spices and lime juice for a delicious yet healthy, savory treat.

SERVES 4

TOTAL TIME: 10 MINUTES

½ cup popcorn kernels

4 teaspoons extra-virgin olive oil

½ teaspoon smoked paprika

½ teaspoon ground cumin

½ teaspoon ground coriander

¼ teaspoon cayenne pepper or to taste

¼ teaspoon salt or to taste

2 teaspoons lime juice or to taste

1. Make the popcorn by combining 2 teaspoons of the olive oil with the popcorn, using your favorite popcorn cooking method, such as a popcorn maker, in the microwave, or on the stovetop.

2. Combine the smoked paprika, cumin, coriander, cayenne pepper, and salt in a small bowl.

3. Pour the hot popped popcorn into a large bowl or bag and top with the remaining 2 teaspoons of olive oil, the lime juice, and the spice mixture. Stir or shake well until all of the popcorn is coated with the seasonings.

Crispy Baked Tofu

Ingredients: Avocado oil spray, one 15-ounce package firm tofu (organic), 1 tablespoon avocado oil, 1 tablespoon gluten-free tamari, 2 tablespoons cornstarch

---

Technique (Convection Oven): Preheat a convection oven to 400°F. Line a baking sheet with parchment paper and lightly coat it with avocado oil spray.

Cut the tofu into ½-inch cubes. Spread the cubes out onto a layer of paper towels and top them with another layer of paper towels. Place a cast-iron skillet or other heavy object on top to help press the liquid out of the tofu.

Remove the skillet after 10 minutes and place the tofu cubes in a bowl with the avocado oil, tamari, and cornstarch. Toss well to coat all of the cubes, lay them on the parchment-lined baking sheet, and bake for 20 minutes, or until golden brown and crispy.

Technique (Conventional Oven): Preheat the oven to 425°F. Line a baking sheet with parchment paper and lightly coat it with avocado oil spray.

Follow the rest of the directions above as written, but check for doneness at about 25 minutes (instead of 20), turning the tofu over halfway through if desired, until golden brown and crispy.

Notes and Storage: To maintain crispiness, it's best to make the tofu right before serving.

The *Best* Tempeh

Tempeh is an excellent plant-based protein that's also a fermented food. However, the tangy taste is not for everyone. Give it a try using this tasty preparation method.

Ingredients: one 8-ounce package (organic) tempeh, optional marinade seasonings (see below), extra-virgin olive oil or avocado oil, salt and pepper to taste

Technique: Steam the tempeh for 5 to 10 minutes. This is optional but preferred, to reduce tempeh's bitterness. Slice the tempeh into thin strips or crumble it. Bring a pot of water with a steamer basket to a boil over high heat. Add the tempeh to the basket and steam for 5 to 10 minutes, until a paring knife or fork can slide through easily, indicating it's tender but still holds its shape. Alternatively, steam the tempeh in the microwave. Drain any excess water.

Marinate the tempeh for 1 hour. This is also optional, but it makes tempeh more flavorful. Depending on the recipe you are adding tempeh to, here are three marinades to try:

- gluten-free tamari, ginger, toasted sesame oil, maple syrup
- lemon juice, parsley, garlic-infused oil, crushed red pepper flakes
- lime juice, avocado oil, oregano, cumin

Cook the tempeh. Heat a large skillet over medium-high heat. Add avocado or olive oil to coat the bottom of the pan. Add the plain or marinated tempeh slices or crumbles. Sauté the tempeh

recipe continues

for 5 to 8 minutes, turning periodically, until lightly browned and crispy. Season with salt and pepper.

Notes and Storage: Store cooked tempeh in an airtight container in the refrigerator for up to 5 days. Tempeh may also be stored in the freezer for 2 to 3 months.

Soft/Medium/Hard-Boiled Eggs

Ingredients: Large (pastured) eggs

Technique: Place cold whole eggs on the bottom of a saucepan and cover with water, 1 inch above the eggs. Heat the saucepan over medium-high heat.

When the water bubbles gently, reduce the heat immediately, allowing a light simmer. Simmer for 10 minutes for hard-boiled eggs, 6 minutes for medium-boiled eggs, and 4 minutes for soft-boiled eggs.

Use a slotted spoon to remove the eggs from the water and gently place them in a bowl of ice water to cool for at least 1 minute before peeling.

Notes and Storage: Soft-boiled and medium-boiled eggs are best eaten immediately. Store hard-boiled eggs in an airtight container in the refrigerator for up to 1 week.

Easy Pan-Seared Salmon

Ingredients: Wild salmon fillets, extra-virgin olive oil or avocado oil, salt and pepper to taste

---

Technique: Heat a large skillet (a cast-iron pan works well) over medium heat. Add olive or avocado oil to coat the bottom of the skillet. Place the salmon fillets, skin side down, and season with salt and pepper. Cook for 4 minutes, flip, and cook for an additional 3 minutes.

Notes and Storage: If using frozen wild salmon, allow it to thaw before cooking. Store extra cooked salmon in an airtight container in the refrigerator for up to 4 days.

Stovetop Shrimp

Ingredients: Extra-virgin olive oil or avocado oil, frozen or fresh shrimp (peeled or unpeeled), salt and pepper to taste

---

Technique: Heat a large skillet (a cast-iron pan works well) over medium heat. Add olive or avocado oil to coat the bottom of the skillet. Place the shrimp in the skillet and season with salt and pepper. Cook for 5 minutes, or until the shrimp become opaque and slightly curled.

Notes and Storage: If using frozen shrimp, allow them to thaw before cooking. Store extra cooked shrimp in an airtight container in the refrigerator for up to 4 days.

EPILOGUE

In the pages of this book, you've discovered the immense power of the gut microbiome—how it can repair and restore the gut barrier, calm the immune system, and reduce inflammation. Yet what you've learned is bigger than simply reducing symptoms or managing disease. This is your story—one where you educate and empower yourself, explore what truly works for you, and have the audacity to try something different in pursuit of better health.

Nature wants to heal. My hope is that the Plant Powered Plus approach has given you the tools, insights, and encouragement to honor your body's innate ability to do just that. Remember, we're not looking for perfection or even an endpoint here—we're embracing a new way of living that is ever evolving and progressing. Regardless of the spark that brought you, you now stand at the threshold of a renewed relationship with yourself and with the life-giving microbes inside you.

This is the "Plus" in Plant Powered Plus: the recognition that vibrant health isn't achieved by food alone. It encompasses the timing of your meals, which supplements you take, the rhythms of your day, the quality of your relationships, your emotional and spiritual well-being, and even how you process old hurts and traumas. Each piece of this puzzle shapes the gut-immune connection, feeding into a steady transformation.

Don't be surprised if your sense of possibility expands. What begins as a dietary change may lead you to deeper introspection, long walks in nature, a spiritual awakening, or heartfelt conversations with people you care about. When you dare to transform your gut, you can't help but open space for something bigger—a lifestyle that heals on many levels.

So here's my invitation to you: Keep going. Carry what you've learned in these pages into every aspect of your life. Keep experimenting, observing, and adjusting. Most importantly, never forget that you possess an astonishing power within you—thirty-eight trillion microbes, working hand in hand with your immune system, all guided by a mind and spirit that can choose to nurture them every single day.

If you feel compelled to share your journey, I would love to hear from you—visit www.theguthealthmd.com or connect with me on social media: @TheGutHealthMD. And if you know someone who could benefit from this book, please share it with them. And thank you for allowing me to be a part of your health journey. It is a tremendous privilege and a dream come true to be able to write books that can change people's lives.

APPENDIX

Medical Conditions Associated with Inflammation & Gut Dysbiosis

AUTOIMMUNE AND ALLERGIC

ANCA-associated vasculitis

Ankylosing spondylitis

Antiphospholipid syndrome

Asthma

Autoimmune hepatitis

Autoimmune pancreatitis

Behcet's disease

Celiac disease

Collagenous colitis

Crohn's disease

Dermatitis herpetiformis

Eczema

Eosinophilic esophagitis

Fibromyalgia

Food allergies

Grave's disease

Guillain-Barré syndrome

Hashimoto's thyroiditis

Interstitial cystitis

Kawasaki disease

Lymphocytic colitis

Multiple sclerosis

Myasthenia gravis

Primary biliary cirrhosis

Primary sclerosing cholangitis

Psoriasis

Psoriatic arthritis

Rheumatoid arthritis

Sarcoidosis

Scleroderma

Seasonal allergies

Sjögren's

Systemic lupus erythematosus

Type 1 diabetes

Ulcerative colitis

HEART, VASCULAR, LUNG, AND GENERAL

Abdominal aortic aneurysm

Aging

Aortic dissection

Aortic valve disease

Atherosclerosis

Atrial fibrillation

Bone density loss

Brain aneurysm

Chronic obstructive pulmonary disease (COPD)

Congestive heart failure

Coronary artery disease

Deep vein thrombosis (DVT)

Endocarditis

Frailty

Low back pain

Myocardial infarction

Myocarditis

Osteoarthritis

Peripheral artery disease

Pulmonary embolism/venous thromboembolism

Pulmonary hypertension

Renal artery stenosis

Rheumatic heart disease

Sarcopenia (muscle loss)

Stroke

Takotsubo cardiomyopathy

Vertebral fractures

APPENDIX

CANCERS

Acute lymphoblastic leukemia (ALL)

Acute myeloid leukemia (AML)

Breast cancer

Cholangiocarcinoma (bile duct)

Chronic lymphocytic leukemia (CLL)

Chronic myelogenous leukemia

Colorectal cancer

Endometrial cancer

Esophageal adenocarcinoma

Esophageal squamous cell cancer

Gallbladder cancer

Glioma (brain cancer)

Hepatocellular (liver) carcinoma

Hodgkin lymphoma

Kidney (renal cell) cancer

Melanoma

Multiple myeloma

Non-Hodgkin lymphoma

Non-small cell lung cancer

Ovarian cancer

Pancreatic cancer

Prostate cancer

Small cell lung cancer

Stomach cancer

Thyroid cancer

HORMONAL

Early menopause

Endometrial hyperplasia

Endometriosis

Erectile dysfunction

Female infertility

Female sexual dysfunction

Hyperthyroid

Hypothyroid

Male hypogonadism (low testosterone)

Male infertility

Menopause

Polycystic ovary syndrome (PCOS)

BRAIN AND PSYCHIATRIC

Alzheimer's dementia

Amyotrophic lateral sclerosis

Anorexia nervosa

Attention-deficit/ hyperactivity disorder

Bipolar disorder

Bulimia nervosa

Chronic fatigue syndrome

Epilepsy

Generalized anxiety disorder

Hepatic encephalopathy

Insomnia

Major depression

Migraine headaches

Neuropathic pain

Parkinson's disease

Post-traumatic stress disorder

Postpartum depression

Premenstrual dysphoric disorder

Restless leg syndrome

Schizophrenia

Vascular dementia

Visceral hypersensitivity

METABOLIC

Acute alcoholic hepatitis

Acute pancreatitis

Alcoholic cirrhosis

Alcoholic steatohepatitis

Chronic kidney disease

Chronic pancreatitis

Gout

Hyperlipidemia

Hypertension

Non-alcoholic fatty liver disease (NAFLD)

Nonalcoholic steatohepatitis (NASH)

Obesity

Type 2 diabetes

FODMAPs

Note: These lists provide a broad overview of low and high FODMAP foods. Some of these foods may be low, moderate, or high in FODMAPs depending on serving sizes. Please note that lists may change as new foods are tested and other foods are retested. Refer to the Monash FODMAP app for the most up-to-date lists of foods, as well as appropriate serving sizes.

Low FODMAP Foods

FRUIT

Avocado (3 slices)	Clementine	Guava (ripe)	Passion fruit	Rhubarb
Banana (small firm)	Coconut (fresh & dried)	Honeydew	Pineapple	Star fruit
Banana chips (dried)	Cranberries (1 Tbsp)	Kiwifruit	Plantain	Strawberries
Blueberries (handful)	Dragon fruit	Lemon	Pomegranate (handful)	Tangelo
Cantaloupe	Grapes	Lime	Raisins (1 Tbsp)	
		Orange	Raspberries	
		Papaya		

VEGETABLES/HERBS

Arugula	Capers	Fennel bulb	Parsnip	Sweet potato (½ small)
Bamboo shoots	Carrots	Gingerroot	Potato (white)	Swiss chard
Basil	Celeriac	Green beans	Pumpkin (canned)	Thyme
Bean sprouts	Chili pepper	Kale	Radish	Tomatoes
Beets (canned or pickled)	Chives	Leek greens	Rosemary	Turnip
Bell peppers	Cilantro	Lettuce	Rutabaga	Water chestnuts
Bok choy	Collard greens	Mint	Scallion (no white part or bulb)	Watercress
Broccoli	Corn (½ cob)	Olives	Seaweed (nori)	Zucchini squash (5–6 slices)
Cabbage (common, red)	Cucumber	Oyster mushrooms	Spinach	
	Eggplant	Parsley	Squash	
	Endive			

BAKING PRODUCTS & BEVERAGES

Cocoa powder	Condiments (mustard, vinegar, soy sauce, ketchup, 1 Tbsp each)	Dark chocolate	Spices	Sugar
		Maple syrup	Starch	Vanilla and almond extract
		Rice syrup	Stevia	

BEVERAGES

Alcohol (white & red wine, beer, gin, vodka, whiskey)	Black tea	Green tea
	Coffee & espresso	Peppermint tea
	Cranberry juice	

LEGUMES

Chickpeas (canned, ¼ cup drained & rinsed)	Edamame (2 handfuls)	Lentils (canned, ½ cup drained & rinsed)	Tempeh
			Tofu (firm)

GRAINS

Buckwheat	Corn tortillas	Polenta	Sourdough wheat breads	Teff flour
Corn flour	Millet	Quinoa		
Corn, fresh (½ cob)	Oats	Rice	Soba noodles	
			Sorghum	

SEEDS

Caraway	Poppy	Pumpkin	Sesame	Sunflower
Chia/flax/hemp				

NUTS

Almonds, almond butter (1 Tbsp)	Chestnuts	Macadamia nuts	Pecans	Walnuts
Brazil nuts	Hazelnuts	Peanuts, peanut butter (2 Tbsp)	Pine nuts	

High FODMAP Foods

FRUCTOSE

Fruit

Apples	Boysenberries	Nashi (Asian pear)	Tinned fruit in natural juice	Most fruit juices
Banana (ripe)	Cherries	Pears		
	Mangoes	Tamarillos	Watermelon	

Sweeteners

Agave	High-fructose corn syrup	Honey

Beverages

Rum

APPENDIX

LACTOSE

Milk

Cow's	Sheep	Custard	Ice cream	Yogurt
Goat's				

Cheeses

Soft, unripened cheeses

FRUCTANS

Vegetables

Artichoke	Cabbage (savoy)	Leeks	Shallots	Sugar snap peas
Asparagus	Eggplant	Okra	Snow peas	
Beetroot (fresh)	Fennel	Onions	Spring onions	
Brussels sprouts	Garlic	Peas		

Grains

Barley	Rye	Wheat

Fruit

Currants	Dried fruit	Grapefruit	Persimmon	Watermelon
Dates				

GALACTANS

Legumes

Baked beans	Broad beans	Lima beans	Silken tofu	Soy milk
Black beans	Fava beans	Navy beans	Soybeans (mature)	Split peas
Borlotti beans	Kidney beans	Pinto beans		

Nuts

Cashews	Pistachios

POLYOLS

Fruit

Apples	Blackberries	Nashi	Pears	Watermelon
Apricots	Cherries	Nectarines	Plums	
Avocados	Lychees	Peaches	Prunes	

Vegetables

Cauliflower	Green bell peppers	Mushrooms (button, portobello, shiitake)	Sweet corn
Celery			

Sweeteners

Isomalt	Mannitol	Sugar-free gum
Maltitol	Sorbitol	Xylitol

Upgrade Your Home

○ Use a high-quality water filter. Consider investing in a reverse osmosis water purification system.

○ Don't buy drinks in plastic bottles.

○ Shift to non-plastic reusables: coffee mugs, water bottles, food containers, straws, kitchen utensils. Bring these with you (such as to the coffee shop).

○ Don't heat food in plastic.

○ All canned food should be BPA-free.

○ Don't buy acidic foods in cans or plastic (sauerkraut, tomatoes).

○ Use loose-leaf tea in stainless steel infusers instead of tea bags.

○ Avoid cling wrap.

○ Wash fresh produce under running water. Consider washing hard produce (apples, pears, peppers, etc.) in DIY natural pesticide remover (1 teaspoon baking soda per 2 cups of water; soak for 12 to 15 minutes, then rinse thoroughly).

○ Switch to organic whole grains, legumes, and soy.

○ Choose organic for thin-skinned plant foods.

○ Upgrade your EVOO game with cold-pressed, high polyphenol varieties.

○ Support sustainable seafood by opting for smaller fish (e.g., sardines, mackerel) or algae-based omega-3 supplements and purchasing seafood from trusted, environmentally conscious sources.

○ Create a friendly sleep environment. Use blackout curtains, a sleep mask, white noise machine, cooler temperatures, and breathable fabrics for optimal sleep.

○ Establish a routine of brushing, flossing, and regular dental cleanings to support the oral microbiome.

ACKNOWLEDGMENTS

Every book starts as an idea, but bringing it fully to life requires the passion, commitment, and talents of many extraordinary people. *Plant Powered Plus* began as my quest to help my patients navigate inflammation and gut health. Witnessing their struggles ignited my desire to create a resource that offers real, practical solutions. This journey has been both challenging and deeply rewarding, and I am incredibly grateful to those who have supported me along the way.

First, my profound gratitude goes to my wife, Valarie. Your constant support, encouragement, and partnership have carried me through every step of this process. Whether I needed clarity, guidance, or just someone to talk things through with, you were always there. The best things I do are always with you.

To my family—Noreen Johnson, Susan and Larry Kobrovsky— your love and unwavering support have shaped my life profoundly. You've always stood by me, creating a foundation that allows me to chase my dreams. I am endlessly grateful to have you by my side.

Dad, I know you're up there. I think of you all the time. Your legacy lives on every time I take my kids camping or canoeing or we watch Syracuse sports. They all have qualities that remind me of you.

Colleen Martell deserves special recognition as my brilliant co-writer, for helping me transform my thoughts into the words you read today. Your patience, creativity, and insight are unmatched.

EA Stewart, your exceptional recipes have brought this book to life, turning nutritional guidance into delicious, practical solutions.

I must thank my amazing publishing team at Avery, particularly Lucia Watson, my editor and trusted guide through our third book together. Lucia, your skill, insight, and thoughtful feedback have elevated this work immeasurably—you're simply the best. Thanks also to Tracy Behar, Lindsay Gordon, Isabel McCarthy, Farin Schlussel, Carla Iannone, Casey Maloney, and Lillian Ball for believing in and supporting my vision.

Stephanie Tade, my literary agent, thank you for your guidance and unwavering belief in my work. You took a chance on me early on, and here we are growing together. Hope you're having as much fun as I am. Thank you to her team, Colleen Martell and Gretchen van Nuys.

I am profoundly thankful to the entire team supporting me behind the scenes—Christina Roberto, Eli Goldstein, Pam Kruusi, Rachel Davis, Amber Ludeman, Matt Silverman, Chiara Kuzmick, Hayley Larsen, Nicole Geer, and many others. Your hard work, creativity, and passion help spread this message and make my work impactful and meaningful.

To my dear friend Simon Hill, my brother from the other side of the world. Thank you for the laughs, the diligent work, and the true friendship. To our incredible team at 38TERA—Kellie Smith, Anna Bearpark, Eden Abagi, and others. Every day is a great day that I get to work with you.

To Chuck Carroll—my dear friend and podcasting partner. Thank you for your friendship and for helping amplify our shared mission.

To the team at ZOE—Jonathan Wolf, Tim Spector, Sarah Berry, Federica Amati, Ali Heston, Rich Willan, and many others through the years—I'm proud of everything we've accomplished together.

My mentors through the years—Drs. Doug Drossman, Nick Shaheen, John Pandolfino, Balfour Sartor, and Peter Kahrilas—thank you for investing in my professional development and helping me grow as a physician and a person.

To my patients and health care colleagues, you are the true inspiration behind *Plant Powered Plus*. Thank you to Kate D'Orazio and the team at The Gut & Microbiome Center for Excellence. To my online community, readers, and members of The Gut Health Collective— your engagement, questions, and commitment to growth fuel my passion for teaching and sharing. Your support means everything.

Thanks to all the podcast hosts, social media friends, journalists, and friends in the media for the support through the years. Thank you to Jon Gresh and the Ivy family for the spiritual leadership that inspires me. I have to thank Brandon Lake and Chris Stapleton for the soundtrack to writing this book.

Finally, my deepest love and gratitude to my children. I am so proud of you, so inspired by you—you are my greatest joy. I love you times infinity.

INDEX